Acute Obstetrics: A Practical Guide

Acute Obstetrics: A Practical Guide

MARTHA C.S. HEPPARD, M.D.
Junior Fellow
American College of Obstetricians and Gynecologists
Kaiser-Permanente
St. Joseph's Hospital
Denver, Colorado

THOMAS J. GARITE, M.D.
Professor and Chairman
Department of Obstetrics and Gynecology
College of Medicine
University of California at Irvine
UCI Medical Center
Irvine, California

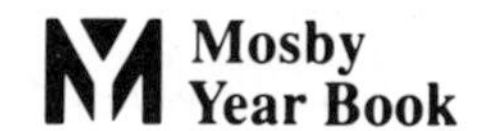

St. Louis Baltimore Boston Chicago London Philadelphia Sydney Toronto

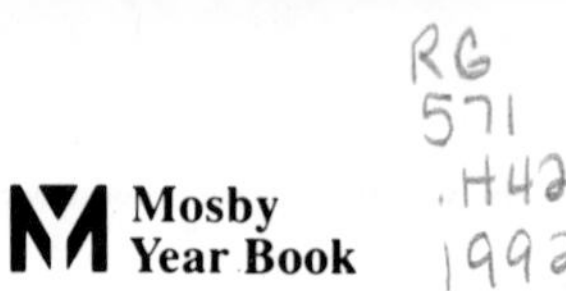

Dedicated to Publishing Excellence

Sponsoring Editor: Stephanie Manning
Assistant Editor: Jane Petrash
Assistant Director, Manuscript Services: Frances M. Perveiler
Production Coordinator: Nancy C. Baker
Proofroom Manager: Barbara Kelly

Mosby–Year Book, Inc., 11830 Westline Industrial Drive, St. Louis, MO 63146

1 2 3 4 5 6 7 8 9 0 CL/ML 96 95 94 93 92

Library of Congress Cataloging-in-Publication Data

Heppard, Martha.
Acute Obstetrics: A Practical Guide / Martha Heppard ; Thomas J. Garite, editor.
p. cm.
Includes bibliographical references and index.
ISBN 0-8016-2147-X
1. Pregnancy, Complications of. I. Garite, Thomas J. II. Title.
[DNLM: 1. Obstetrics—methods—handbooks. 2. Pregnancy Complications—handbooks. 3. Risk Factors—handbooks. WQ 39 H529h]
RG571.H42 1991 92-28052
618.3—dc20 CIP
DNLM/DLC
for Library of Congress

NOTICE

Every effort has been made to ensure that the drug dosage schedules herein are accurate and in accord with the standards accepted at the time of publication. However, as new research and experiene broaden our knowledge, changes in treatment and drug therapy occur. Therefore, the reader is advised to check the product information sheet included in the package of each drug he plans to administer to be certain that changes have not been made in the recommended dose or in the contraindications. This is of particular importance in regard to new or infrequently used drugs.

To my twin sons, Matthew and Patrick, who made it possible for me to experience a high risk pregnancy and gave me 3 months of bedrest to write this book

FOREWORD

As an intern rotating through medicine, I remember my reliance on the *Washington Manual of Medical Therapeutics*. It was my security blanket, and although it weighed down my already burdened white coat, I felt naked without it. When I began my rotations through obstetrics there was no similar guide, but I felt no void. Since the information and technology explosion of the 1970s and 1980s, however, I have concluded that a similar need now exists for our students and house officers, especially those newly exposed to obstetrics. A handy manual that gives the necessary background and the hows and whys of commonly seen problems in obstetrics would seem to be a priceless reference to carry and use.

Dr. Heppard perceived this need when she originally wrote and distributed her "Intern's Survival Guide." Because so many who saw and used this tool have encouraged her to make it more widely available, we embarked on putting it into its present format. *Acute Obstetrics: A Practical Guide* has been updated and made more comprehensive, to cover all acute problems encountered by new physicians, nurse practitioners, or midwifes based at the hospital or prenatal clinic. More importantly, we have diligently attempted to make this a manual which is not encumbered by regional biases and prejudices so that it can, as much as possible, be employed in all institutions in all regions. Differences will exist nonetheless, and we have tried to point out where they are likely to occur. It has been a pleasure and a privilege to participate with Dr. Martha Heppard on this project, and I hope that you who use it will find it the useful resource that we intended.

Thomas J. Garite, M.D.
Professor and Chairman
Department of Obstetrics and Gynecology
College of Medicine
University of California Irvine
UCI Medical Center
Irvine, California

PREFACE

This book provides the practicing physician, resident, and medical student with a quick and accurate reference concerning the management of high risk obstetric patients. The management schemes described here are based on the most recent literature and standard practices to which I, as a resident, was exposed at the Department of Obstetrics and Gynecology at the University of California Irvine (UCI) Medical Center. Although patient management varies from hospital to hospital, this book provides fundamental information upon which treatment may be initiated.

The book fills a void in reference material supporting the management of high risk obstetric patients. At the beginning of my internship I found myself relying on notes scribbled on sheets of paper and scattered handouts to develop management schemes for patient care. Researching through texts and current literature proved to be too time consuming in an acute care scenario. This book provides patient care guidelines for residents and other physicians who labor under similar time constraints.

I first distributed an abbreviated version of this book as an informal guide in 1988 and found that it was well received by my fellow residents and other physicians associated with UCI Medical Center. In addition to being a quick and practical reference, I was told by practicing physicians that they found the guide useful in reviewing for Ob/Gyn boards. Medical students and residents commented that the guide was an extremely valuable tool in providing quality patient care.

I would like to thank Dr. Thomas J. Garite, Chairman of the Department of Obstetrics and Gynecology, Lanie M. Adamson, Senior Editor in the department, the department staff, and my fellow residents for their help and encouragement which made it possible to transform my informal guide into this book. I also want to thank the publisher, Mosby–Year Book, for its patience and support.

Martha C.S. Heppard, M.D.

CONTENTS

Part I

EVALUATION OF THE PATIENT

PRENATAL EVALUATION 1

I. Background. Prenatal care is one of the few routine examples of regularly provided preventive health care commonly accepted in Western medicine. From a cost-benefit standpoint, prenatal care is most effective at lowering perinatal mortality and morbidity. It accomplishes this goal by identifying pregnant women and their fetuses at increased or high risk for specific adverse outcomes, and applying appropriate diagnostic and therapeutic measures. The purposes and goals of prenatal care include:

A. Prevention of perinatal morbidity and mortality
B. Application of other preventive health measures not specifically related to pregnancy but instituted because the patients are now in the health care system (i.e., Pap smears, tuberculosis skin testing)
C. Provision of appropriate psychosocial counseling
D. Patient education and preparation
E. Contraceptive planning

II. Contributors to Perinatal Mortality. Since reduction of perinatal mortality and morbidity is the most realistic goal, the physician must first be aware of the main contributors to such adverse outcome and then be able to assess the risk for these specific contributors.

A. Antepartum Fetal Death

1. Etiology
    a. Uteroplacental insufficiency
    b. Fetal anomalies
    c. Cord accidents
    d. Abruptio placentae

e. Hydrops fetalis
f. Fetal infections
2. Prevention
a. Risk assessment
b. Ultrasound and genetic testing
c. Antepartum fetal testing

B. **Intrapartum Fetal Death.** This is now rare, due largely to routine electronic or frequent auscultative fetal heart rate monitoring in labor.

C. **Neonatal Death**
1. Etiology
a. Prematurity (accounts for the vast majority)
b. Asphyxia
c. Anomalies
d. Infections
2. Prevention
a. Risk identification
b. Education and detection of early premature labor

III. Prenatal Evaluation

A. **History.** Eighty percent of all antenatal high-risk factors are identified on the **first visit.**
1. **History of Present Illness**
a. Ascertain the state of the woman's present health and well-being.
b. Identify any pregnancy complications that occurred before the first visit.
c. **Accurate dating** may be accomplished by evaluating the patient's:
1) Menstrual history
2) Uterine size on the first prenatal examination
3) Fetal ultrasound
4) Gestation at which fetal heart tones were first detected by Doppler echocardiography and fetoscopic examination
5) Quickening date
2. **Past Obstetric History**
a. Place special emphasis on:
1) Complications of previous pregnancies
2) Size of previous babies
3) Course of previous labors and deliveries
b. Other past medical and surgical history

3. **Family History**
   a. Place emphasis on:
      1) History of genetic diseases/anomalies
      2) Obstetric problems
      3) Diabetes
      4) Hypertension
   b. Other significant family history
4. **Social History**
   a. How is the pregnancy welcomed, wanted, and perceived?
   b. How is the pregnancy impacting the family emotionally and economically?
   c. What are the plans for future pregnancies and contraception?
   d. Use of illicit drugs and alcohol
   e. Occupation and impact of pregnancy
   f. Support of family and friends
   g. Other
5. **Review of Systems.** This is generally limited to likely current problems (i.e., morning nausea) and is directed at any actual positive past medical history.

B. Physical Examination

1. Routine complete physical examination
2. Size and location of pregnancy
3. Establish fetal viability (fetal heart tones [FHTs])
4. Pelvic measurements to determine the likelihood of a successful vaginal birth
5. **Initial Laboratory Assessment** (Table 1–1)

IV. Initial Problem List. After the initial history, physical, and laboratory assessment, the patient's initial problem list can be constructed. Problems should include:

A. Intrauterine pregnancy with excellent/good/fair/poor dates at ______ weeks' gestation

B. Diagnosis-Based Problems

1. Hypertension
2. Diabetes
3. Others

C. Identified Risk Factors

V. Identifying Risk Factors. Since 80% of all antenatal high-risk patients are identified on the first visit, this is the best

TABLE 1–1.
Initial Laboratory Assessment

1. CBC
2. Urinalysis
3. Screening test or routine culture for urinary tract infection
4. Venereal Disease Research Laboratory or rapid plasma reagin testing
5. Blood type, Rh, antibody screen
6. Hepatitis B surface antigen
7. Rubella titer
8. Pap smear
9. Population-dependent routine tests
   a. Purified protein derivative
   b. Vaginal/cervical culture for chlamydial infection and gonorrhea
10. One-hour post glucola for patients at risk for diabetes (Only patients at risk will have screening at the initial visit in addition to the routine screening of all patients at 28 weeks.)
    a. Family history of diabetes
    b. Maternal age >25
    c. Glucosuria
    d. Marked obesity
    e. Accelerated fetal growth
    f. Polyhydramnios
    g. History of:
       1) Macrosomic baby
       2) Baby with a congenital anomaly
       3) Preeclampsia
       4) Previous gestational diabetes
       5) Previous stillborn
       6) Polyhydramnios

time to identify patients at risk for the three major factors that contribute to perinatal mortality.

A. Risk Factors for Perinatal Death Due to Hypoxia/Asphyxia

1. Diabetes
2. Hypertension (chronic and pregnancy induced)
3. Post dates
4. Collagen vascular disease
5. Previous stillbirth
6. Chronic renal disease
7. Chronic hypoxia
   a. Pulmonary origin
   b. Cardiac origin

8. Severe anemia
9. Thyrotoxicosis
10. Intrauterine growth retardation

B. Risk Factors for Perinatal Death Due to Prematurity

1. Multiple gestation
2. Previous premature birth
3. Two or more midtrimester abortions
4. Teenager ($<$17 years of age)
5. In utero diethylstilbestrol exposure
6. Uterine malformation
7. Cervical cerclage/cervical incompetence
8. Uterine fibroids
9. Polyhydramnios
10. Thyrotoxicosis
11. Acute infections or other acute medical illnesses, such as:
    a. Hepatitis
    b. Pyelonephritis
12. Abdominal surgery with this pregnancy
13. Premature contractions ($\geq$5 per hour)
14. Previous cervical cone biopsy
15. Cervical dilatation $>$2 cm
16. Vaginal bleeding

C. Risk Factors for Anomalies and Genetic Diseases

1. Race
    a. Southeast Asian—α-thalassemia
    b. Ashkenazi Jews—Tay Sachs disease
    c. Mediterranean—β-thalassemia
    d. Black
        1) Sickle cell disease
        2) Glucose-6-phosphate dehydrogenase deficiency
2. Advanced maternal age—trisomies
3. Advanced paternal age—new autosomal dominant mutations
4. Family history of genetic disease or multifactorial birth defect
5. Previous pregnancy with birth defect or genetic disease
6. Teratogen exposure (TORCH: toxoplasmosis, other [viruses], rubella, cytomegalovirus, herpes [simplex viruses] infections)
7. Diabetes
8. Elevated or low maternal serum α-fetoprotein

9. Polyhydramnios or oligohydramnios
10. Intrauterine growth retardation

VI. Follow-Up Prenatal Care

A. The majority of problems that appear after the first prenatal visit but before hospital admission will be picked up by monitoring the following:
1. Routine blood pressure
2. Routine fundal height
3. Simple history for new patient problems (i.e., "Any problems?")
4. Ultrasound (Because ultrasound has become nearly routine, many unexpected problems will be identified on a sonogram.)

B. Routine Follow-Up Visits for Low-Risk Patients
1. **First Visit.** Initial history, physical, laboratory assessment, and problem list development as described previously.
2. **Subsequent Visits**
   a. Frequency
      1) Every month until 26 to 28 weeks
         a) If no FHTs are detected with use of Doppler echocardiography on the first visit, the patient should return more frequently until FHTs are documented.
         b) At 18 to 20 weeks, FHTs should be detectable with fetoscopic examination. If not, the patient should return every 1 or 2 weeks until they are heard.
      2) Every 2 to 3 weeks until 36 weeks' gestation
      3) After 36 weeks, every week until term
   b. At each visit review the patient's problem list and obtain her:
      1) Weight
      2) Blood pressure
      3) Urine for sugar and albumin levels
      4) Fundal height
      5) FHTs
      6) Fetal presentation after about 32 weeks
      7) New complaints
   c. Follow-up laboratory assessment
      1) Maternal serum α-fetoprotein at 16 weeks

2) One-hour post glucola (diabetes screen) at 28 weeks
3) For all Rh-negative patients at 28 weeks:
   a) Repeat the antibody titer.
   b) Administer RhoGAM if the antibody titer test results are negative.
4) Repeat a CBC at 28 weeks in all patients.

d. Topics for Discussion. At some time during the entire prenatal course, discuss each of the following with your patient.
   1) Weight gain
   2) Diet
   3) Exercise
   4) Sexual activity
   5) Common complaints of pregnancy
   6) Explanation of any risk factors
   7) Toxin and teratogen avoidance
      a) Smoking
      b) Alcohol
      c) Drugs of pregnancy
   8) Travel during pregnancy
   9) Signs and symptoms of toxemia
   10) Signs and symptoms of premature labor
   11) Prenatal classes
      a) Prenatal/Lamaze method
      b) Baby care
      c) Cesarean birth
      d) Breast feeding
   12) Fetal movement counting
   13) Labor and delivery instructions
      a) When to come in
      b) Where to go
   14) Anesthesia
   15) Contraception/sterilization
   16) Breast and bottle feeding
   17) Choice of pediatrician
   18) Circumcision

INTRAPARTUM EVALUATION

2

When a pregnant patient is admitted to the hospital because of antepartum complications, it is vital that the condition of mother and fetus be thoroughly documented. The admission note serves as the cornerstone for future treatment and care. Because of its importance, this note may be quite complex and may detail many problems. The following example demonstrates a complete evaluation in a format that is clear and easy to read.

ADMISSION NOTE

I. Date and Time________________________

II. History of Present Illness

- Mrs/Miss ____(name)____ is a (age, nationality, gravida, para, aborta), with (number) living children.
- Her last menstrual period (LMP) was on (date).
- Her estimated date of confinement is (date), placing her estimated gestational age at (weeks).
- She presented to the obstetric emergency room with complaints of ______________. (If she was transported from another hospital, give the name of the hospital from which she was transported and the reason for transport.)
- Provide a brief paragraph of the history of her present illness. Use the problem list to fill in details of labor status, i.e., preterm labor.

III. Problem List

- **Problem # 1. Intrauterine Pregnancy**
  - LMP (date) Estimated gestational age (weeks).
  - Her menses were (regular/irregular).

- She is (sure/unsure) of her LMP.
- Oral contraceptive pills were (taken/not taken) within the 3 months preceding conception.
- Her first urine pregnancy test was on (date).
- Her first examination was on (date) at (weeks' gestation). Her uterine size was/was not appropriate for her gestational age.
- She has had (number) follow-up examinations. Size = Dates? (Y/N).
- A sonogram performed on (date and at what gestational age) revealed (list all parameters measured and their equivalency in weeks).
- Her fundal height is (cm) and fetal heart tones in beats per minute are (rate).
- Therefore her estimated gestational age = (weeks), by (poor/fair/good/excellent) dates.

- **Problem #2. Primary Reason for Admission.** Example: Preterm labor (PTL)
  - Briefly detail her history (uterine contractions, dysuria, fever).
  - If she was transported from another hospital, describe her medical course prior to admission at your hospital (i.e., tocolysis with magnesium sulfate ($MgSO_4$) for (hours).
  - Explain the current status of her labor, her pertinent physical examination (cervix, fundal firmness), and laboratory findings (CBC with differential, urinalysis, cervical and amniotic fluid cultures, and Gram's stain).

IV. Past Medical History

Detail the patient's illnesses, operations, allergies, and medication use. Provide her obstetric history (date, place, method of termination if an abortion occurred or was performed, gestational age, weight, route of delivery if pregnancy progressed to viability, prenatal problems, complications).

V. Family History

Inquire especially into the patient's family history of hypertension, diabetes mellitus, twins, congenital anomalies, and genetic diseases.

VI. Social History

Determine the patient's use of tobacco, alcohol, prescribed and nonprescribed drugs. Does the patient have a stable marriage? Is there evidence of social problems? Has she planned for contraception or sterilization postpartum?

VII. Review of Systems

Limit to pertinent positives only.

VIII. Physical Examination

- Vital signs (include weight)
- Head/eyes/ears/nose/throat, funduscopic examination (especially important for patients with diabetes mellitus and hypertension)
- Throat, lungs, breast, heart
- Abdominal examination
  - Fundal height
  - Contraction frequency, duration, strength
  - Fetal position on Leopold's maneuver
  - Estimated fetal weight
- Pelvic examination (to be done on all patients **except for those with third trimester bleeding, patients in whom placenta previa has not yet been ruled out, and those with premature rupture of membranes**
- Perform a sterile speculum examination on patients with premature rupture of membranes and third trimester bleeding
- Extremities (edema, tenderness)
- Neurologic examination—deep tendon reflexes

IX. Laboratory Evaluation/Diagnostic Data

- Include prenatal laboratory examinations in addition to those tests ordered during this admission.
- Determine uterine and fetal heart rate monitoring patterns.

X. **Assessment.** Example: Patient with PTL

- Intrauterine pregnancy at ______ weeks' gestation
- PTL
- Other problems

XI. Plan. Example: Patient with PTL

- Bed rest
- Induce tocolysis with $MgSO_4$, then attempt to wean to oral terbutaline (or obtain consent for a study protocol. (Always check updated study lists at your institution to see if the patient is eligible.)
- Laboratory tests: CBC with differential, serum electrolytes (if indicated), urinalysis with culture and sensitivity, cervical/vaginal/perineal swab for Gram's stain and group B β-streptococcus culture, cervical culture for *Neisseria* gonorrhoeae.________________________

Signature

Part II

MEDICAL COMPLICATIONS OF PREGNANCY

ACUTE ABDOMINAL PAIN 3

The diagnosis of acute abdominal pain in pregnancy is challenging to the obstetrician, internist, and general surgeon. The maternal physiologic and anatomic changes during pregnancy affect the patient's symptoms, signs, and laboratory parameters during an acute illness. Many common causes of acute abdominal pain may be associated with increased maternal and fetal morbidity and mortality if not treated early in the disease process. The following discussion focuses on the more common causes unrelated to the gestation.

ACUTE APPENDICITIS

I. Background

A. **Definition.** Inflammation of the vermiform appendix.

B. **Incidence.** Approximately 1 in 2,000 pregnancies (unchanged from the general population). The frequency of appendicitis is constant through all trimesters.

C. **Perinatal Morbidity and Mortality.** The fetal loss rate is 15%. Abortion and preterm labor are increased, especially in the presence of peritonitis, particularly with a ruptured appendix.

D. **Maternal Morbidity and Mortality.** The maternal mortality rate is 2.0% in the first trimester and rises to 7.3% in the third trimester. The mortality rate in a nonpregnant patient is less than 0.1% for uncomplicated acute appendicitis and 5% when perforation has occurred.

II. Evaluation

A. **History.** A history of anorexia, nausea, vomiting, and right-side abdominal pain is usually present.

B. **Physical Examination.** Perform a thorough physical. With appendicitis, the patient may have a fever and will most often but not always demonstrate abdominal tenderness (Table 3–1), guarding, and rebound. Figure 3–1 illustrates the usual position of the appendix throughout pregnancy.

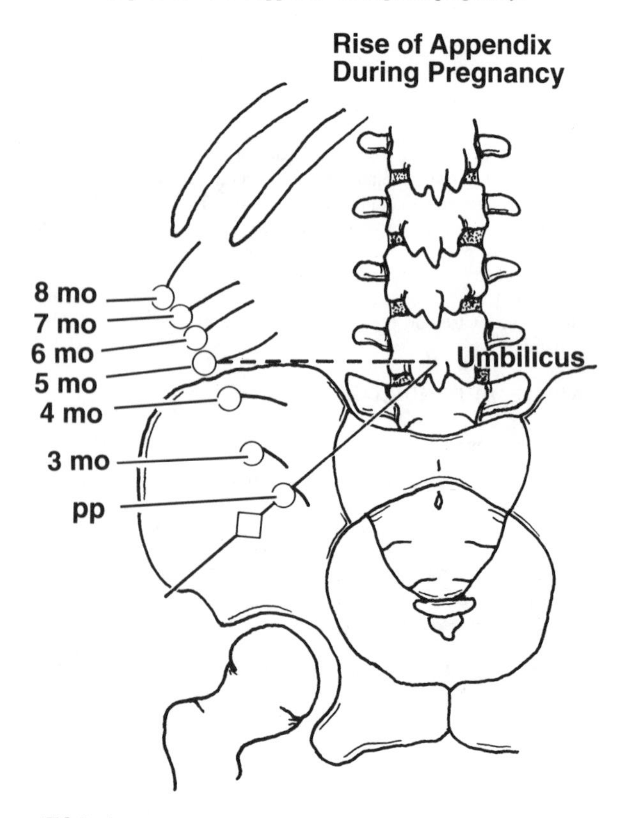

FIG 3–1.
Schematic representation of the location of the appendix during pregnancy in relationship to McBurney's point. (Redrawn from Baer JL, Reis RA, Arens RA: JAMA 1932; 98:1359.)

TABLE 3–1.
Comparison of Findings in Pregnant and Nonpregnant Patients With Appendicitis*

	Pregnant	Nonpregnant
Diagnostic accuracy	72%	75%
Symptoms	Nausea, vomiting, increased frequency of urination, abdominal pain, anorexia	
Physical findings	Abdominal pain (100%) First trimester: right lower quadrant (100%) Second trimester: right lower quadrant (80%) Third trimester: right upper quadrant (20%)	Abdominal pain (100%) Right lower quadrant (65%) Pelvis (30%) Flank (5%)
	Rebound tenderness (75%)	Present
	Guarding (60%)	Present
	Fever >100.2° (18%)	High 100.4°
Laboratory findings		
White blood cell count	Normal pregnancy: 12,500–16,000 per mm^3 with 80% bonds	Normal WBC 3,000–10,000 per mm^3 Most patients demonstrate a shift to the left. Not all demonstrate leukocytosis. Fewer than 4% have a normal WBC and no shift to the left.
Urinalysis	Pyuria is present if the ureter or renal pelvis is in contact with the inflamed appendix	Pyuria: Rare

*From DeVore GR: *Clin Perinatol* 1980; 7:349–369. Used by permission.

C. **Diagnostic Data.** Obtain a CBC, with differential (a left shift of the WBC is usually present), and a urinalysis (pyuria may be present with appendicitis).

D. **Diagnosis.** This diagnosis is often difficult to make in pregnancy.

1. The presenting symptoms of acute appendicitis mimic the

common symptoms of early pregnancy (anorexia, nausea, vomiting).
2. As the gestation advances, the appendix moves upward and laterally in the abdomen (see Fig 3–1).
3. The leukocytosis commonly seen with acute appendicitis is normally present during pregnancy.
4. During pregnancy the abdominal signs of appendicitis are often atypical of those noted in a nonpregnant patient.

E. Differential Diagnosis

1. Pyelonephritis is the diagnosis most commonly confused with acute appendicitis, especially as pregnancy progresses. Bacteriuria is present with pyelonephritis but absent in appendicitis.
2. Other disorders that may present with similar findings include a ruptured ovarian cyst/corpus luteum, ovarian torsion, preterm labor, abruptio placentae, degenerating myoma, cholecystitis, pneumonia, and, rarely, appendiceal endometriosis.
3. When undiagnosed appendicitis stimulates preterm labor, after delivery the contracted uterus may disrupt a previously walled-off infection, spilling purulent material into the abdomen and creating a surgical abdomen postpartum.

III. Therapeutic Management (Table 3–2)

A. Surgical intervention is mandatory. A vertical midline incision between the symphysis pubis and umbilicus, or right paramedian incision, provides adequate exposure for removal of the appendix or treatment of other gynecologic disorders that mimic appendicitis. The preoperative diagnosis of appendicitis is correct less than half the time.

B. Cesarean section should be avoided in the presence of appendicitis unless absolutely necessary.

C. Antibiotics are unnecessary in uncomplicated appendicitis. When gangrene or perforation occurs, antibiotics directed against bowel flora are indicated.

D. Postoperatively, observe the patient on labor and delivery for at least the first 24 hours. If contractions occur, consider tocolysis, depending on the gestational age and the patient's status. If the patient has septic complications, she may be unable to tolerate the cardiovascular and hemodynamic side effects of some tocolytic agents.

TABLE 3–2.
Recommendation of Surgical Approach in Pregnant Patients With Appendicitis*

Surgical Technique	Uncomplicated	Gangrenous	Perforated
Bury stump if possible	X		
Double ligate stump	X	X	X
Close all layers with nonabsorbable suture	X	X	X
Do not place suture in subcutaneous fat	X	X	X
Irrigate wound with antibiotics	X	X	X
Close skin with locking mattress suture	X		
Leave skin and subcutaneous tissue open		X	X
Place intraabdominal drain			X

*From DeVore GR: *Clin Perinatol* 1980; 7:349–369. Used by permission.

CHOLELITHIASIS AND CHOLECYSTITIS

I. Background

A. Definitions

1. **Cholelithiasis** is the presence of gallstones.
2. **Cholecystitis** is inflammation of the gallbladder.

B. Etiology. Cholesterol crystals retained in the gallbladder may form stones (gallstones), subsequently obstruct the cystic duct, and result in inflammation of the bladder wall. When repeated episodes of acute inflammation occur, the gallbladder may become chronically infected and develop edematous, rigid walls.

C. Incidence

1. **Asymptomatic gallstones** are identified in 2%–4% of women undergoing a routine obstetric ultrasonic examination.
2. **Acute cholecystitis** occurs in 1 of 1,000 pregnancies.
3. Pregnancy is thought to increase the prevalence of gallstones by:
   a. Progesterone-mediated decrease in gallbladder emptying.

b. Increasing cholesterol saturation in the bile (resulting from the 50% increase in esterified and free cholesterol in the bloodstream).

c. The decreasing bile salt pool may result in a relative cholesterol excess, thus leading to gallstone formation.

4. In the general population, 2% of patients with previously silent gallstones develop symptoms. This figure is thought to be unchanged in pregnancy.

II. Evaluation

A. History. The symptoms of cholecystitis are the same as in the nonpregnant patient. The patient will usually complain of anorexia, nausea, vomiting, and pain of abrupt onset (usually lancing, occasionally deep and cramping), originating in the midportion of the epigastrium, radiating to the upper right area of the abdomen or back. The pain may be colicky or steady for up to an hour.

B. Physical Examination. Although one third of nonpregnant patients with cholecystitis have a palpable gallbladder, this is found in less than 5% of pregnant patients. Localized tenderness may suggest pancreatitis or abscess formation around the gallbladder, while rebound may suggest perforation.

C. Diagnostic Data

1. Obtain a CBC with differential, amylase, and an alkaline phosphatase level. If the alkaline phosphatase level is not elevated above that found in normal pregnancy, consider obtaining specific alkaline phosphatase isoenzymes, 5′ nucleotidase, in addition to blood and urine samples for an amylase:creatinine clearance ratio (Fig 3–2).
2. **Ultrasound** evaluation of the gallbladder demonstrates stones in 96% of patients in whom acute cholecystitis has been diagnosed clinically.
3. **Cholescinctigraphy** (technetium-99m creates a minimal radiation exposure for the fetus) has excellent sensitivity and specificity in the diagnosis of cholecystitis. This is the diagnostic procedure of choice in a nonpregnant patient, and may be used during pregnancy when the benefits are thought to outweigh the risks.

D. The diagnosis of cholecystitis may be difficult to make in pregnancy because:

1. Anorexia, nausea, and vomiting are commonly seen in the first trimester of pregnancy.

$$C_{AM}/C_{CR}\ \% = \frac{\text{Amylase Clearance}}{\text{Creatinine Clearance}} \times 100$$

$$C_{AM}/C_{CR}\ \% = \frac{\dfrac{\text{(Amylase) Urine} \times \text{(Volume)* Urine}}{\text{(Amylase) Serum}} \times \text{Time*}}{\dfrac{\text{(Creatinine) Urine} \times \text{(Volume)* Urine}}{\text{(Creatinine) Serum}} \times \text{Time*}} \times 100$$

$$C_{AM}/C_{CR}\ \% = \frac{\text{Amylase Urine}}{\text{Amylase Serum}} \times \frac{\text{(Creatinine) Serum}}{\text{(Creatinine) Urine}} \times 100$$

FIG 3–2.
Formula for calculating the amylase/creatinine clearance ratio (*volume and time cancel). (From DeVore GR: *Clin Perinatol* 1980; 7:349–369. Used by permission.)

2. A moderate leukocytosis (which is usually found with this disorder) is often present during pregnancy.
3. Alkaline phosphatase is produced by the placenta and elevated in uncomplicated pregnancies.

E. The **differential diagnosis** includes hepatitis (severe acute viral versus alcoholic), duodenal ulcer perforation, acute pancreatitis, pyelonephritis, appendicitis, pneumonia, and myocardial infarction.

III. Therapeutic Management

A. Medical management is successful in the majority of patients, and thus an initial attempt at conservative management should be made. This therapy consists of:

1. Intermittent nasogastric suction
2. Intravenous colloids
3. Narcotics for pain control
4. Antibiotics if evidence of sepsis is present, or if the patient does not respond to conservative therapy within 4 days

B. Surgical management is necessary when at initial presentation the patient has a surgically "acute" abdomen and when medical management fails. The second trimester is the optimal period in which to perform surgery because the uterus is below the operative field and thus at decreased risk for abortion or preterm labor. When surgery is indicated, the rate of maternal and fetal morbidity and mortality increases with delay.

C. Asymptomatic gallstones are not to be removed surgically during pregnancy.

ACUTE PANCREATITIS

I. Background

A. **Definition.** Inflammation of the pancreas.

B. **Incidence.** Acute pancreatitis occurs in 0.01%–0.1% of pregnancies (the incidence in nonpregnant patients is 0.5%). While this disorder is seen in all trimesters, it is more frequent in the third trimester and postpartum.

C. **Pathophysiology.** Pancreatitis arises from pancreatic autodigestion by enzymes that are inappropriately activated by alcohol abuse, gallstones, infection, ischemia, trauma, vasculitis, hyperlipidemia, and hypercalcemia. Alcohol abuse and gallstones are thought to be associated with 80% of cases of acute pancreatitis in nonpregnant patients. In pregnancy, in the majority of cases the disease is thought to be related to **gallstones.** It is usually self-limiting, and resolves within a week when medically managed.

D. **Perinatal Morbidity and Mortality.** Abortion and preterm labor may be triggered by disease complications such as hypovolemia, hypoxia, and acidosis.

E. **Maternal Morbidity and Mortality.** Maternal mortality in mild and moderate pancreatitis is unchanged from that noted in uncomplicated pregnancies. When severe pancreatitis develops, the mortality is greater when managed medically than when managed surgically.

II. Evaluation

A. **History.** Elicit information regarding the risk factors detailed in the previous section. The patient may complain of severe midepigastric pain radiating through to her back, as well as nausea, vomiting, and fever.

B. **Physical Examination.** A thorough physical examination may reveal fever and confirm the presence of midepigastric pain or tenderness radiating posteriorly.

C. Diagnostic Data

1. Obtain a CBC with differential, serum amylase, lipase, glucose, electrolyte panel (include creatinine, calcium, magnesium, and phosphorus); urine (spot sample) amylase and creatine.
2. Amylase and lipase levels are elevated with this disease (and other gastrointestinal and reproductive tract disorders), but this change may be masked by the normal elevation of amylase (up to fourfold its normal value) in midpregnancy. Serial amylase and lipase values may be helpful in diagnosing pancreatitis. The magnitude of the values does not correlate with disease severity. When these values remain elevated longer than 1–2 weeks, a pancreatic pseudocyst or ascites may be developing.
3. An **amylase:creatinine clearance ratio** may assist in this diagnosis. It is elevated with this disease, and remains elevated after the acute rise of serum amylase, which occurs within the first 2 days of acute pancreatitis. The ratio is 1%–4% in a healthy nonpregnant patient and 2.0%–3.5% in uncomplicated pregnancies. The ratio of serum amylase to creatinine is decreased compared with that in the nonpregnant state as a result of the increased creatinine clearance during pregnancy (see Fig 3–2).
4. **Hypocalcemia** is commonly present and can be corrected with IV calcium gluconate.
5. **Hyperglycemia** may be present. Consider administration of regular humulin insulin, depending on the severity of the patient's condition.
6. An **ultrasonic examination** or **computed tomographic** scan may assist in diagnosis when the patient's presentation or recovery is atypical.

D. Differential Diagnosis. Acute cholecystitis, perforated ulcer, renal colic, dissecting aortic aneurysm, pneumonia, vasculitis complicating a connective tissue disorder, intestinal obstruction, and diabetic ketoacidosis.

III. Therapeutic Management

A. Mild and Moderate Pancreatitis

1. **Nasogastric suction** (to avoid stimulation of the pancreas) and intravenous hydration are mandatory until the patient is improved symptomatically and biochemically (usually 3–5 days). When improved, she may receive a clear liq-

uid diet and then gradually advanced during the next 2 days to regular food.

2. **Meperidine** (Demerol), 75–100 mg IM every 4 hours, may be administered for pain relief.
3. **Antibiotics** are indicated only if infection develops (i.e., ascending cholangitis or pancreatic abscess).
4. **Avid monitoring of vital signs, fluid intake and output, and electrolytes** is necessary because some degree of third spacing and dehydration occurs in each patient. The need for large fluid replacement coincident with hypotension and respiratory insufficiency indicates worsening disease and a necessity for surgical intervention.
5. **Complications.** Pancreatic pseudocysts occur in 2%–10% of patients. These may be complicated by pancreatic ascites, abscess development, hemorrhage and rupture, or pleural effusion.

B. **Severe Pancreatitis.** Mild and moderate disease may worsen despite conservative medical management. Surgical intervention is necessary in the event of:

1. **Cardiovascular Collapse or Respiratory Insufficiency.** In these cases, either a wide sump drain may be placed, or peritoneal lavage via a laparotomy incision may be performed to remove the toxic exudate from the pancreas.
2. Common bile duct obstruction with **cholangitis.**
3. **Pancreatic abscess.**
4. Life-threatening **hemorrhagic pancreatitis.**

PEPTIC ULCER DISEASE (PUD)

I. Background

A. **Definition.** A peptic ulcer is the defect in the mucosa of the esophagus, stomach, or duodenum caused by gastric acid.

B. **Incidence.** PUD occurs in 5% of the population and is quite rare in pregnancy.

C. **Etiology.** An increase in stomach secretion of hydrochloric acid and pepsin may initiate or maintain an ulcer. Disease improvement may be seen in pregnancy because of the elevated level of progesterone, which results in decreased gastric acid production and increased gastric mucous secretion. In addition, the placenta produces plasma histaminase, which inactivates, or blocks the effect of, histamine (an activator of hydrochloric acid secretion).

D. Perinatal and Maternal Morbidity and Mortality. Mild and moderate PUD has morbidity and mortality rates equivalent to those in uncomplicated pregnancies. When an indication for surgery is present, medical management results in a 44% mortality rate (maternal and fetal) and surgical management in a 13% maternal and 26% fetal mortality rate. The mortality rate from PUD in the general population is 2–5 per 100,000 people per year.

II. Evaluation

A. History. The patient may complain of moderate to severe midepigastric pain (boring, burning, or cramping) lasting for 15–60 minutes. The pain is often relieved by ingesting food or antacids, and exacerbated by alcohol, aspirin, or coffee. If the lesion is in the pyloric region (or if several ulcers are present elsewhere), vomiting may occur. Complaints of hematemesis or melena signify erosion of blood vessels at the ulcer base.

B. Physical Examination. A complete examination is often significant only for minimal tenderness in the midepigastric region.

C. Diagnostic Data. Serum electrolytes, liver enzymes, and CBC with differential are usually at normal levels. If iron deficiency anemia is present, it may be a result of poor dietary intake of iron, or of gastrointestinal bleeding (if hematemesis or melena is present).

D. Differential Diagnosis. The differential diagnosis for this disorder includes acute pancreatitis, chronic cholecystitis, and acute appendicitis.

E. PUD is so infrequent in pregnancy that when newly diagnosed causes such as cancer or Zollinger-Ellison syndrome must be considered.

III. Therapeutic Management

A. Mild Disease

1. Patients with uncomplicated PUD are instructed to refrain from gastric acid stimulants. In addition, they are encouraged to avoid late night snacks to prevent gastric acid stimulation during sleep.

2. **Antacids**
   a. Magnesium hydroxide, calcium carbonate, and aluminum hydroxide may all be safely used during pregnancy (Table 3–3). Sodium bicarbonate may cause fluid retention and cardiac disease.
   b. Recommended dosage is 80 mEq magnesium hydroxide, calcium carbonate, or aluminum hydroxide 1 hour after meals and every 1–2 hours thereafter, with 160 mEq at bedtime.
3. **Histamine analogs** should be utilized.
   a. **Famotidine** (Pepsid), 40 mg orally daily at bedtime (or 20 mg twice daily). After ulcer improvement, the dosage may be decreased to 20 mg daily.
   b. **Ranitidine hydrochloride** (Zantac), 150 mg orally twice daily (or 300 mg daily at bedtime).
   c. **Cimetidine hydrochloride** (Tagamet), 800 mg orally daily at bedtime, or 300 mg four times a day (with meals and at bedtime), or 400 mg twice a day.
4. **Anticholinergics** are used infrequently. They may provide relief to patients who are unresponsive to antacids, and in patients who have epigastric pain during the night. The most frequently used anticholinergic is propantheline bromide (Pro-Banthine). It is administered in a 15 mg tablet orally 30 minutes before each meal, and two tablets (30 mg) at bedtime.

TABLE 3–3.
Antacids and Their Characteristics*

Ingredient	Characteristics
Sodium bicarbonate	Rapid and potent neutralizer; yields large absorbable sodium; may induce milk alkali syndrome
Magnesium hydroxide	Slow but prolonged action; poorly absorbed; osmotic laxative; serum magnesium must be monitored in renal insufficiency
Calcium carbonate	Potent neutralizer; causes constipation; may produce hypercalcemia, milk alkali syndrome, or late acid rebound
Aluminum hydroxide	Slow; not very potent; causes constipation; absorbs phosphate and some drugs

*From DeVore GR: *Clin Perinatol* 1980; 7:349–369. Used by permission.

5. Sedation with **phenobarbital** may be required during an acute episode of discomfort.

B. Peptic ulcer complications are rare in pregnancy.

1. When **bleeding** occurs from the ulcer base,
   a. **Initiate treatment** with
      1) Nasogastric suction
      2) Cold isotonic saline lavage
      3) Blood replacement
   b. Obtain a **gastroenterologist** consultation and consider utilizing the following diagnostic and therapeutic procedures:
      1) **Diagnostic endoscopy** to localize the bleeding vessel (90% accuracy), with possible electrocoagulation (90% successful) of the bleeding site
      2) **Selective angiography** with **embolization** of the affected vessel
         a) This will expose the fetus to radiation.
         b) Maternal complications include liver and stomach necrosis.
   c. When the patient is severely ill and has lost 30% or more of her blood volume within 12 hours, **vagotomy, pyloroplasty, or partial gastrectomy** may be indicated.
2. Patients with **luminal obstruction** require continuous nasogastric suction for a minimum of 3 days. If the patient does not respond within this time, a surgical drainage procedure (i.e., pyloroplasty with vagotomy) may be required.
3. Ulcer **perforation** during pregnancy mandates immediate surgical treatment. If managed conservatively, maternal mortality approaches 100%.
4. When surgical treatment is necessary during the third trimester, document fetal maturity and consider concurrent cesarean section to allow improved visualization of the upper area of the abdomen and to avoid fetal distress resulting from hypotension that may occur during the procedure.

PYELONEPHRITIS

See Urinary Tract Infections.

BIBLIOGRAPHY

DeVore GR: Acute abdominal pain in the pregnant patient due to pancreatitis, acute appendicitis, cholecystitis, or peptic ulcer disease. *Clin Perinatol* 1980; 7:349–369.

Kammerer WS: Nonobstetric surgery in pregnancy. *Med Clin North Am* 1987; 71:551–559.

Landers D, Carmona R, Crombleholme W, et al: Acute cholecystitis in pregnancy. *Obstet Gynecol* 1987; 69:131–133.

Lowe TW, Cunningham FG: Surgical diseases complicating pregnancy, in Cunningham FG, MacDonald PC, Gant NF (eds). *Williams Obstetrics,* ed 18, suppl 3. Raritan, NJ, Ortho Pharmaceutical, December/January, 1990.

ASTHMA 4

I. Background

A. Definition. Asthma is a disorder in which paroxysmal dyspnea occurs in the presence of spasmodic bronchial contractions. Wheezing is common.

B. Etiology. Asthma may have an allergic or idiosyncratic cause, with overlap between these categories.

1. **Allergic**
    a. Includes one-third of all asthmatics and a higher proportion of pregnant asthmatics.
    b. Serum IgE levels are elevated.
    c. Positive skin reactions and positive responses to provocative tests (airborne allergens, exercise, emotional stress) are noted.
    d. A family history of asthma is frequently present.
2. Idiosyncratic
    a. Includes two-thirds of **all** asthmatics, and a smaller proportion of pregnant asthmatics.
    b. Serum IgE levels are normal.
    c. Provocative and skin test results are negative.

C. Incidence

1. Asthma is present in 0.4%–1.3% of pregnancies.
2. Status asthmaticus occurs in 0.05%–0.2% of pregnancies.

D. Perinatal Morbidity and Mortality

1. Perinatal mortality is unchanged from that noted in uncomplicated pregnancies.
2. The only fetal complication is an increased incidence of intrauterine growth retardation, which is attributed to hypoxemia in the mother, with resultant hypoxemia in the fetus. Intrauterine growth retardation occurs exclusively in those patients with severe disease and in those whose disease has not been properly treated.
3. An infant born to an asthmatic mother has a 5%–7% risk of

developing asthma during the first year of life, and a 58% risk of developing it during his or her lifetime.

II. Evaluation

A. **History.** Assess the severity of the attack. Has the patient been hospitalized previously for asthma? Needed corticosteroids? Been intubated? How does the patient compare this attack with previous attacks? Were there any precipitating factors? Has she been compliant with her medications?

B. **Physical Examination**

1. Evaluate whether the patient is using accessory muscles in her breathing effort. Agitation or somnolence indicates decompensation.
2. Vital signs consistent with a severe episode include a pulse greater than 120 beats/min, respirations more than 30/min, and a pulsus paradoxus more than 18 mm Hg.
3. Perform a complete physical examination, and pay special attention to the airway. The intensity of wheezing does not correlate with the severity of the asthma. Rule out upper and lower respiratory infections.

C. **Differential Diagnosis.** Asthma usually is not difficult to diagnose, especially with a good history and physical examination. The differential diagnosis includes:

1. Left ventricular failure
2. Pulmonary embolism
3. Upper airway obstruction (tumor, edema)
4. Chronic bronchitis
5. Pneumonia
6. Dehydration

D. **Diagnostic Data**

1. **Arterial blood gases (ABGs)** are useful in evaluating the severity and chronicity of an attack. Mild hypoxemia and mild respiratory alkalosis are present early in an asthmatic attack. Metabolic alkalosis occurs gradually, and with a severe, prolonged attack, muscle exhaustion produces respiratory acidosis (Tables 4–1 and 4–2).
2. **IMPORTANT: If the patient's pCO_2 is high, she is in respiratory failure and may need endotracheal intubation and mechanical ventilation.**
3. **Pulmonary function tests** are very useful to assess the severity of the attack and the degree of improvement with treatment. Spirometry may be performed at the bedside to

TABLE 4–1.
Acid-Base Balance and Blood Gases*

	Nonpregnant	Pregnant
PO_2 (mm Hg)	98–100	101–104
PCO_2 (mm Hg)	35–40	25–30
Arterial pH	7.38–7.44	7.40–7.45
Bicarbonate (mEq/liter)	24–30	18–21
Base deficit (mEq/liter)	0.07	3–4

*From Gleicher N (ed): *Principles of Medical Therapy in Pregnancy.* New York, Plenum Medical Book Co, 1985. Used by permission.

TABLE 4–2.
Metabolic and Respiratory Acidosis and Alkalosis*

The primary acid-base disturbances result from conditions that initially affect the HCO_3^- (metabolic acidosis and alkalosis) or from states that initially alter the PCO_2 (respiratory acidosis and alkalosis). Each of these primary disturbances causes the blood pH (H^+ concentration) to shift **away** from normal by changing the ratio of $PCO_2/[HCO_3^-]$ and evokes compensatory responses that return pH **toward** but not completely to normal.

1. **Metabolic acidosis** results from a reduction in HCO_3^- that reflects the accumulation of nonvolatile acids. The compensatory response is increased ventilation, leading to a fall in PCO_2.
2. **Metabolic alkalosis** occurs from a primary increase in the HCO_3^-. The compensatory response is hypoventilation, causing a rise in PCO_2.
3. **Respiratory acidosis** is the result of insufficient pulmonary removal of CO_2 (increased PCO_2) leading to an increase of H_2CO_3. The compensatory response is an increase in renal recovery and generation of HCO_3^-, leading to a rise in serum HCO_3^- concentration.
4. **Respiratory alkalosis** occurs due to hyperventilation (decreased PCO_2). The compensatory response is increased renal HCO_3^- loss and reduced regeneration, leading to a fall of serum HCO_3^- concentration.

	Primary change	**pH**	**Compensatory response**
Metabolic acidosis	$\downarrow HCO_3^-$	↓ pH	$\downarrow PCO_2$
Metabolic alkalosis	$\uparrow HCO_3^-$	↑ pH	$\uparrow PCO_2$
Respiratory acidosis	$\uparrow PCO_2$	↓ pH	$\uparrow HCO_3^-$
Respiratory alkalosis	$\downarrow PCO_2$	↑ pH	$\downarrow HCO_3^-$

Metabolic acidosis results from accumulation of fixed (nonvolatile) acid (due to ingestion, endogenous production) or from loss of alkali.

*From Orland MJ, Saltman RJ: *Manual of Medical Therapeutics.* Boston, Little, Brown, 1986. Used by permission.

measure the volume of air expired in the first second of expiration (FEV_1). This value, expressed as a percentage of forced vital capacity (FVC), exceeds 75% in normal patients. When this ratio declines below 30%, severe disease is present and hospitalization is indicated (Tables 4–3 and 4–4 and Fig 4–1).

4. **Chest x-ray** is useful to rule out conditions that may be exacerbating the asthma. Asthmatic lungs often demonstrate hyperinflation.
5. Obtain a **sputum** sample and examine it for eosinophils, white blood cells, bacteria, and Charcot-Leyden crystals.
6. Obtain serum for a CBC with differential and an electrolyte panel.

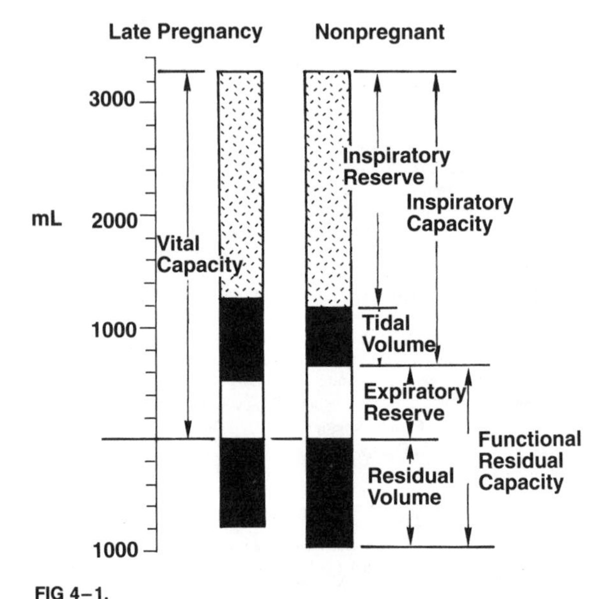

FIG 4–1.
Lung volume and capacities in pregnancy. (From Hytten FE, Leitch I: *The Physiology of Human Pregnancy*, ed 2. Oxford, Blackwell Scientific, 1971, p 120. Used by permission.)

TABLE 4–3.

Lung Volumes and Capacities*

Test	Definition	Change in Pregnancy
Respiratory rate	—	No significant change
Tidal volume	The volume of air inspired and expired at each breath	Progressive rise throughout pregnancy of 0.1–0.2 L. In late pregnancy the tidal volume is probably 40% greater than before conception and mixes with a (functional) residual volume nearly 20% smaller, a change making for greatly increased efficiency of gas mixing
Expiratory reserve volume	The maximum volume of air that can be additionally expired after a normal expiration	Lowered by approx. 15% (0.55 L in late pregnancy compared to 0.65 L post partum). The increased depth of respiration takes place at the expense of the expiratory reserve
Residual volume	The volume of air remaining in the lungs after a maximum expiration	Falls considerably (0.77 L in late pregnancy compared to 0.96 L post partum, a fall of approx. 20%)
Vital capacity	The maximum volume of air that can be forcibly inspired after a maximum expiration	Unchanged except for possibly a small terminal diminution
Inspiratory capacity	The maximum volume of air that can be inspired from the resting expiratory level	Increased by approx. 5%
Functional residual capacity	The volume of air in the lungs at the resting expiratory level	Lowered by approx. 18% (see remarks under tidal volume)
Minute ventilation	The volume of air inspired or expired in 1 min	Increased by approx. 40% as a result of the increased tidal volume and unchanged respiratory rate (10.34 L in late pregnancy compared to 7.27 L postpartum)

*From Main DM, Main EK: *Obstetrics and Gynecology. A Pocket Reference.* St Louis, Mosby–Year Book, 1984. Used by permission.

TABLE 4–4.
Tests of Respiratory Function*

Test	Definition	Change in Pregnancy
Maximum voluntary ventilation (maximum breathing capacity)	The maximum minute ventilation attainable by voluntary hyperventilation	Unchanged
Timed vital capacity	The proportion of the vital capacity that can be expired in the first second	Unchanged
Diffusing capacity	The rate at which a gas passes from the alveoli into the blood at a partial pressure difference of 1 mm Hg	Unchanged (measured with CO)
Airway resistance	Resistance to flow in the airways	Reduced. Both mean and maximum flow rates are unaltered, but the pressure required to achieve these is less

*Adapted from Hytten FE, Lind T: *Diagnostic Indices in Pregnancy.* Basel, Ciba–Geigy, 1973, p 27; as published in Main DM, Main EK: *Obstetrics and Gynecology. A Pocket Reference.* St Louis, Mosby–Year Book, 1984. Used by permission.

III. Therapeutic Management. In general, this is the same whether the patient is or is not pregnant.

A. Provide **oxygen** at 2–3 L/min by nasal cannula. Maintain the po_2 above 60 mm Hg.

B. **Hydrate** the patient with 5% dextrose in water at 100–200 ml/hr.

C. If this is an acute attack, administer:

1. **Aerolized Bronchodilator**
   a. **Metaproterenol (Alupent),** 0.3 ml in 2.5 ml normal saline by nebulized inhaler. If neither subcutaneous terbutaline nor epinephrine is used, this may be repeated every 2 hours for three total doses and then every 4–6hours, **or**
   b. **Isoetharine (Bronkosol),** 0.5 ml in 2.5 ml normal saline, by nebulized inhaler every 2–4 hours, **or**
   c. **Metaproterenol** (Alupent) and **isoetharine** (Bronkosol) may be alternated every 2 hours for three total doses.

d. **Parenteral Sympathomimetics**

1) **Terbutaline** should not be used to initiate treatment because of its delayed onset of action (30–60 minutes). It has a longer serum half-life than epinephrine, and, therefore, may be used for long-term treatment. It may be administered subcutaneously in a0.25 ml dose. The dose may be repeated once in 20 minutes. (Hold for a pulse >115 beats/min.)
2) **Epinephrine** may be utilized in place of terbutaline. It is also administered subcutaneously, but the dose is 0.3–0.5 ml of a 1:1,000 dilution. The dose may be repeated every 30 minutes (hold for a pulse >115 beats/min) up to three times to achieve a symptomatic response. Relative contraindications (as with terbutaline) are severe hypertension and cardiac disease.
3) **Aminophylline** (80% theophylline) may be given, in addition to terbutaline (as severity warrants), in a loading dose of 5–6 mg/kg intravenously for a period of 20–30 minutes, and then followed by a continuous infusion of 0.9 mg/kg/hr. If the patient has taken oral theophylline intermittently, decrease her loading dose by half (measure the theophylline level and adjust accordingly).
   The therapeutic theophylline plasma concentration is 10–20 μg/ml. Serious complications may arise if the theophylline level exceeds 30 μg/ml. Side effects of aminophylline include anorexia, nausea, vomiting, nervousness, and headache. The theophylline half-life is shortened in cigarette smokers.
4) **Glucocorticoids. Do not hesitate to administer these to a pregnant patient if an indication for their use is present.**
   a) **Methylprednisolone** (Solu-Medrol) may be administered in a loading dose of 2 mg/kg intravenous push (IVP). The average loading dose is 120 mg and maximum is 200 mg.
   b) Follow the loading dose with a maintenance dose of Solu-Medrol. Frequently used regimens include:
      i) 0.75 mg/kg (average dose 40 mg) **IVP** every 4 hours.
      ii) 60 mg **IVP** every 6 hours.

c) After 2–3 days, Solu-Medrol may be discontinued and **oral prednisone** initiated at 30 mg twice daily, with gradual tapering by 5 mg every other day, beginning with the evening dose.

d) **Hydrocortisone** (Solu-Cortef) may be used instead of Solu-Medrol. The relative IV strengths are 4:1 (Solu-Medrol:Solu-Cortef).

e. **Antibiotics** are not routinely used unless a bacterial infection is strongly suspected.

f. If the patient responds to emergency treatment with metaproterenol and parenteral sympathomimetics, she may be discharged home with an **Alupent** inhaler (two puffs every 4–6 hours) and continuation of **theophylline** (if previously prescribed). Have the patient return to your office within 1 week (sooner if symptomatic) to reevaluate her theophylline level and pulmonary function.

g. If the patient requires aminophylline, glucocorticoids, or antibiotics, consider admitting her for further treatment and observation.

D. **Chronic management** in pregnant patients is similar to that of nonpregnant patients. The goal is to optimize pulmonary function and prevent acute attacks.

1. **Educate** the patient and her family so that they will understand the disease and avoid precipitating factors (exercise, cold, dust, animal dander, tartrazine, aspirin, nonsteroidal anti-inflammatory agents) and will seek care early in an attack.
2. **Bronchodilators** are useful in controlling mild asthmatic attacks.
   a. Aerosolized agents such as **Alupent** and **Bronkosol** are usually the first line of therapy and are taken two–four times daily, as indicated, for rapid resolution of mild exacerbations.
   b. **Terbutaline,** 2.5–5 mg orally three times a day, and **theophylline,** 200–400 mg orally twice daily, may be used when inhalants no longer control the attacks.
   c. Hepatic clearance of theophylline during the third trimester of pregnancy is decreased by 20%–30% in comparison with the nonpregnant state. Thus, theophylline levels must be monitored periodically.
3. **Corticosteroids** may be used in those patients with frequent severe attacks despite bronchodilator treatment.

   a. Do not hesitate to use steroids in pregnant patients if they are indicated. The risks associated with maternal hypoxia are greater than those with steroid use.
   b. Consider using **beclomethasone,** two puffs (100 μg) four times daily.
4. If clinically indicated, **cromolyn sodium** may be used prophylactically for patients with asthma induced by exercise and cold. The usual dosage is 20 mg (one capsule) via aerosol inhaler (e.g., Intal inhaler) four times daily. Experience with cromolyn sodium in pregnancy is limited.

E. Delivery

1. The vaginal route is preferable.
2. An epidural anesthetic is the one of choice.
3. If the patient is taking steroids for a long time period, increase these to stress doses (25 mg Solu-Medrol **IVP** or 100 mg Solu-Cortef **IVP**). Gradually taper the steroids postpartum as described in section IIIC1d(4).

BIBLIOGRAPHY

Creasy RK, Resnik R: *Maternal-Fetal Medicine*. Philadelphia, WB Saunders, 1984.

Orland MJ, Saltman RJ: *Manual of Medical Therapeutics*. Boston, Little, Brown, 1986.

Wyngaarden JB, Smith LH: *Cecil's Textbook of Medicine,* ed 17. Philadelphia, WB Saunders, 1985.

DIABETES 5

I. Background

A. **Definition.** Diabetes mellitus (DM) is a metabolic disorder of carbohydrate intolerance, usually caused by insufficient insulin secretion or inadequate insulin activity. Alterations in carbohydrate, fat, and protein metabolism during pregnancy may exacerbate current diabetes or uncover latent diabetes.

B. **Incidence.** Insulin-dependent (type 1) diabetes occurs at a rate of 0.1%–0.5% in the general population. The incidence of gestational diabetes (classes A_1 and A_2 as defined in Table 5–1) is 3%–12% of pregnancies. These account for 90% of patients with diabetes complicating pregnancy.

C. **Etiology.** Patients >25 years of age, markedly obese, with glucosuria, accelerated fetal growth, or a history of macrosomia, anomalous fetus, stillbirth, family history of diabetes, preeclampsia, previous gestational diabetes, previous stillbirth, or polyhydramnios, are at high risk of developing diabetes during pregnancy. One or more of these risk factors are present in almost half of the patients who develop gestational diabetes.

1. Screen high-risk patients for diabetes at their initial prenatal care visit.
2. At 28 weeks screen all other patients, plus those high-risk patients whose first screen results were within normal range.
3. Screen with a 1-hour post glucola, in which glucose (50 g) is ingested orally and a venous blood specimen is drawn 1 hour later.
   a. The screen is within normal limits if the plasma glucose level is ≤140 mg/dL (sensitivity 80%, specificity 90%).

TABLE 5–1.
White's Classification of Diabetes in Pregnancy*

	Pregestational Diabetes			
Class	Age of Onset (yr)	Duration (yr)	Vascular Disease	Therapy
A	Any	Any	0	A-1, diet only A-2, insulin
B	>20	<10	0	Insulin
C	10-19 or	10-19	0	Insulin
D	10 or 20		Benign retinopathy	Insulin
F	Any	Any	Nephropathy	Insulin
R	Any	Any	Proliferative retinopathy	Insulin
H	Any	Any	Heart disease	Insulin

	Gestational Diabetes		
Class	Fasting Glucose Level		Postprandial Glucose Level
A-1	<105 mg/dl	and	<120 mg/dl
A-2	≥105 mg/dl	and/or	≥120 mg/dl

*From *ACOG Technical Bulletin* 1986: 92:May. Used by permission of the American College of Obstetricians and Gynecologists.

b. If >140 mg/dL, obtain a 3-hour glucose tolerance test (GTT). Approximately 15% of these patients will have an abnormal GTT.

4. A normal GTT is defined as:
   a. Fasting blood sugar (FBS) ≤105 mg/dL
   b. 1-hour plasma glucose ≤190 mg/dL
   c. 2-hour plasma glucose ≤165 mg/dL
   d. 3-hour plasma glucose ≤145 mg/dL
5. Gestational DM is present if two of the three GTT plasma glucose values (excluding the FBS) exceed the normal range.

D. White's classification of diabetes in pregnancy is the most commonly used system (Table 5–1).

E. Perinatal Morbidity and Mortality

1. Perinatal mortality is 2%–5%. Intrauterine fetal death occurs at an increased rate in insulin-dependent diabetics.

2. The increased rate of malformations seen in insulin-dependent diabetics is believed to correlate with poor control of diabetes.
   a. Most malformations noted in infants of diabetic mothers occur during the first 7 weeks of pregnancy (Table 5–2).
   b. Diabetic women who require insulin have a 6%–8% chance of delivering an infant with a major malformation, 2–4 times the rate in the general population. Class A_1 diabetics do not have an increased rate of fetal anomalies.
3. Fetal macrosomia in insulin-dependent diabetics increases the risk of birth trauma.

TABLE 5–2.

Congenital Malformations in Infants of Diabetic Mothers*

Cardiovascular
Transposition of the great vessels
Ventricular septal defect
Atrial septal defect
Hypoplastic left ventricle
Situs inversus
Anomalies of the aorta
Central nervous system
Anencephaly
Encephalocele
Meningomyelocele
Microcephaly
Skeletal
Caudal regression syndrome
Spina bifida
Genitourinary
Absent kidneys (Potter syndrome)
Polycystic kidneys
Double ureter
Gastrointestinal
Tracheoesophageal fistula
Bowel atresia
Imperforate anus

*From Gabbe SG, Niebyl JR, Simpson JL (eds): *Obstetrics: Normal and Problem Pregnancies.* New York, Churchill Livingstone, 1986, p 902. Used by permission.

4. Additional neonatal complications include hypoglycemia, hyperbilirubinemia, hypocalcemia, polycythemia, and transient respiratory distress.
5. Decreased neonatal and perinatal morbidity, particularly macrosomia and hypoglycemia, are seen when maternal metabolic variation is minimized.

F. Maternal Morbidity

1. Ten percent of Class A_1 insulin-dependent diabetics will progress to Class A_2 during the current pregnancy.
2. All insulin-dependent diabetics are at risk of developing vascular disease, with specific involvement of the eyes (retinopathy, macular edema), kidneys, heart, and extremities.
3. The rate of preeclampsia rises in diabetic patients.
4. Infection and dehydration may precipitate diabetic ketoacidosis **(DKA).**
5. Hypothyroidism is a frequent finding in diabetic patients during pregnancy.

II. Evaluation

A. History. Elicit information regarding the patient's previous pregnancies (history of macrosomia, stillbirth, insulin use), history of polyuria, vaginitis (*Candida* infections are seen more frequently in diabetic patients), results of screening tests, and GTTs.

B. Physical Examination. Particular attention needs to be directed to the patient's vital signs (evaluate her blood pressure carefully since pregnancy-induced hypertension is more common in diabetic patients), funduscopic examination, fundal height (size >dates?), and neurologic examination (especially the vibration sense in extremities, which is the most sensitive test for detecting neuropathy).

III. Diagnostic Evaluation

A. Laboratory studies indicated for all diabetic patients include:

1. Plasma blood sugar (BS) (Any random BS >200 mg/dL is diagnostic for diabetes.)
2. Baseline CBC with differential
3. Electrolyte panel

4. Clean-catch urinalysis with culture and sensitivity (avoid catheterization in diabetic patients in the absence of pyelonephritis)
5. Consider obtaining a 24-hour urine collection for protein and creatinine clearance if your patient has an elevated creatinine or class F DM.
6. See Antepartum Testing.

B. **Additional evaluations indicated for classes A_2, B, C, D, E, and F:**
1. EKG for patients with vascular or renal disease
2. Thyroid panel
3. Genetic counseling
4. Hemoglobin A_{1c}
5. Ophthalmologic examination

IV. Therapeutic Management

A. Therapeutic management depends on diagnostic data. The following discussion does not apply to patients in diabetic ketoacidosis (DKA), who require more aggressive management. If the patient is in DKA, refer to a standard medical textbook or obtain consultation from an internist or perinatologist.

B. **American Diabetic Association (ADA) Diet**
1. Adherence to the ADA diet is important for therapeutic success in all patients with diabetes.
2. The ADA recommends that 30 calories per kilogram actual body weight (2,200–2,400 calories) be consumed as 45% carbohydrate, 20% protein, and 35% fat.
3. Calorie intake should be balanced throughout the day: 25% breakfast, 30% lunch, 30% dinner, and 15% bedtime snack.
4. Instruct patient to eat all of her meals.

C. **Insulin Administration**
1. If the patient's disease is **newly diagnosed as class A_1 or A_2** diabetes, and if her fasting BS is between 105 and 125 mg/dL, recommend an ADA diet for one week; then reexamine her FBS. If her FBS is >105 mg/dL, start her on a regimen of insulin therapy.*
2. Calculate the patient's **24-hour insulin dosage** accord-

*Some authorities advocate routine insulin therapy for class A_1 diabetes.

ing to trimester. Modifications may be made if this is the first time the patient has been on insulin (decrease dosage) and if the patient is markedly obese (increase dosage).

a. First trimester: 0.6 unit of insulin per kilogram body weight
   Second trimester: 0.7 unit of insulin per kilogram body weight
   Third trimester: 0.8 unit of insulin per kilogram body weight
b. The 24-hour insulin requirement is **divided into morning and evening injections,** with all insulin administered subcutaneously 20–30 minutes before meals. When ordering insulin, specify **human** insulin (i.e., Humulin [Lilly]). Human insulin (made by monoclonal techniques), is purer than that obtained from other sources such as pork.
   1) **Morning:** Administer ⅔ of the total daily dose as follows:
      a) Two-thirds NPH (neutral protamine Humulin insulin; peaks in 6–8 hours)
      b) One-third regular (regular Humulin insulin; peaks in 2–4 hours)
   2) **Evening:** Administer one third of the total daily dose as follows:
      a) One-half NPH
      b) One-half regular
c. Frequently, a **three-dose regimen** is employed: NPH ± regular insulin at breakfast, regular with dinner, and NPH at bedtime. An **alternative for new borderline class A_2 diabetics** is to treat with a single dose of NPH in the morning. In an attempt to normalize blood sugars throughout the day, 20 units of NPH is a good starting dose. If the patient is obese, a larger dose may be required. If the FBS remains greater than 105 mg/dL, give additional NPH at bedtime.

D. If her **FBS is <250 mg/dL** and she is spilling no or minimal ketones, manage her disease as an outpatient, with insulin and outpatient education.

E. If her **FBS is >250 or she is spilling a moderate or large amount of ketones** (or if both conditions exist), consider admission, including inpatient education and continuous insulin infusion.

1. If the patient has a moderate or large amount of ketones, check her **venous bicarbonate** level.
   a. If indicative of acidosis, examine her serum **acetone** level and arterial blood gas.
   b. **The diagnosis of DKA includes:**
      1) Plasma glucose >300 mg/dL
      2) Plasma bicarbonate <15 mg/dL
      3) Serum acetone positive at a 1:2 dilution
      4) Arterial pH <7.30
   c. During pregnancy, DKA may develop with hyperglycemia as mild as 200–300 mg/dL.
   d. If the patient has DKA, obtain a medical or perinatal consultation.
2. **Hydrate** your patient with 1 L of normal saline (NS) infusing at 200 mL/hr. Follow this with NS into which 30 mEq KCl/L has been added. Infuse at 125 mL/hr.
3. **Continuous Insulin Infusion:** Place 50 units of regular Humulin insulin into 500 mL of NS. Start the infusion at a rate appropriate for the patient (for example 3 units (30 mL/hr). Continue the infusion for approximately 1 day, adjusting the dosage and drip rate as needed.
4. Capillary glucose testing should be performed every 2 hours. You (or the house officer) are to be notified of all values.
5. Check patient's urine at each void for sugar and acetone.
6. When changing to subcutaneous insulin therapy, calculate the patient's total 24-hour insulin requirement by adding the hourly amounts of IV insulin infused on the previous day. Use this as a starting point to calculate appropriately divided subcutaneous doses.

F. **All patients on subcutaneous insulin are to have:**
   1. **Capillary glucose testing** every day before breakfast, lunch, dinner, and bedtime snack. Therapeutic objectives are for maternal plasma glucose values to be in the range of those seen in nondiabetic pregnant patients (Table 5–3).
   2. **Urine** examined for **sugar** and **acetone** at each void.

G. **Make insulin adjustments as follows:**
   1. If the serum glucose level is elevated, increase the insulin dose as detailed below.

TABLE 5–3.
Normal Plasma Glucose Values During Pregnancy

Meal Status	Range (mg/dL)	Maximum (mg/dL)
Fasting	60–90	105
Before lunch, dinner, and bedtime snack	60–105	120
2 hours' postprandial	120	135

If elevated before:	Then increase:
Breakfast	Evening NPH
Lunch	Morning regular
Dinner	Morning NPH
Bedtime snack	Evening regular

NOTE: The patient receives an evening snack with the ADA diet. Note the number of meals and snacks that the patient is actually eating, and whether friends and family are bringing extra food to your patient.

2. Increase insulin by 20% to a maximum of 4 units at a time.
3. If the FBS is persistently high despite increased insulin, obtain a capillary glucose test at 2 A.M. to rule out the possibility of rebound hyperglycemia.

V. Antepartum Surveillance*

A. Class A_1 (uncomplicated, without any other indications for antepartum testing)

1. Weekly FBS
2. Dietary counseling
3. Ultrasound to rule out macrosomia at 37–38 weeks
4. Begin weekly contraction stress testing (CST) at 40 weeks' gestation.

B. Classes A_2 and B

1. Weekly FBS in the office. Home capillary glucose testing after each meal and at bedtime.
2. Dietary counseling

*Antepartum surveillance of diabetic patients with contraction stress testing (CST) may not be utilized at your institution. A reasonable alternative may be the twice-weekly biophysical profile (BPP). Amniotic fluid volume may not be a reliable predictor of fetal status in diabetic patients because of their propensity toward polyhydramnios.

3. Ultrasound for gestational dating upon admission; then in the second trimester at approximately 20 weeks to rule out fetal anomalies.
4. CST and nonstress testing (NST):
   a. At 32 weeks, begin weekly CSTs and NSTs. Run NSTs between CSTs, so that testing is performed every 3–4 days.
   b. Earlier testing (25–28 weeks) is indicated in patients with proteinuria, intrauterine growth retardation, or hypertension.

C. Classes D, E, and F

1. Begin antepartum testing as detailed for Classes A_2 and B, but begin at 26–28 weeks
2. Deliver at 38 weeks, or sooner in the presence of **intrauterine growth retardation, pregnancy-induced hypertension,** or abnormal test results.

VI. While the patient is antepartum, discuss sterilization. Special consents may be required in the antepartum period depending on state laws.

VII. On Discharge Home (Antepartum)

A. Be sure your patient has all the necessary prescriptions and equipment and that she fully understands her dietary and insulin instructions.

B. She must be seen weekly in the office. (Have blood drawn for an FBS upon her arrival each week.)

C. Patients should be scheduled for antepartum testing as discussed in section V above.

VIII. For Diabetic Patients in Labor at Term, or Those in Whom Labor Is Being Induced (Table 5–4)

A. Patients in whom labor is to be induced should have **documented fetal lung maturity,** unless delivery is being undertaken for maternal indications. In addition to routine labor care, **capillary glucose testing is performed every 2 hours** if values are normal and stable; otherwise every 1 hour. Glucose values should be maintained at 80–110 mg/dL.

B. Induction patients are to be **NPO after midnight** the night before the induction is to begin. Instruct your patient to

TABLE 5–4.

Bishop Score for Inducibility of Labor*

Factor	Score 0	Score 1	Score 2	Score 3
Cervical dilatation (cm)	Closed	1–2	3–4	5+
Cervical effacement (%)	0–30	40–50	60–70	80+
Fetal station	−3	−2	−1.0	−1. +2
Cervical consistency	Firm	Medium	Soft	
Cervical position	Posterior	Midposition	Anterior	

Range of scores = 0–13. Prerequisites: Multiparity, gestation of at least 36 wk, vertex presentation, and with a normal past and present obstetric history. Predictions: Patients with scores of 9 or more will have safe, successful inductions with an average length of labor of less than 4 hr.[1] Modifications of this score to make it applicable to more patients and improve predictability:[2]

Add one point for:	*Subtract one point for:*
Pre-eclampsia	Postdatism
Totally elective	Nulliparity
Each prior vaginal delivery	Premature or prolonged ROM

Predictive Value

Score	
Score: 0–4	45–50% failure rate
5–9	10% failure rate
10–13	0% failure rate

Selected references: 1. Bishop EH: Pelvic scoring for elective induction. *Obstet Gynecol* 1964; 24:266.
2. Hughey MJ, McElin TW, Bird CC: An evaluation of preinduction scoring systems, *Obstet Gynecol* 1976; 48:635.

*From Main DM, Main EK: *Obstetrics and Gynecology. A Pocket Reference.* St Louis, Mosby–Year Book, 1984. Used by permission.

continue her capillary glucose testing but to **omit** her **bedtime and morning insulin.** Instruct your patient to arrive at labor and delivery early in the morning.

C. Some patients will require an **insulin infusion** (i.e., patients who require prolonged inductions and those whose diabetes is not controlled on intermittent subcutaneous insulin doses). Start your patient on Ringer's lactate solution (LR) at a minimum of 125 mL/hr. Check her urine for ketones at each void. If ketones are present, place her on D5LR (dextrose 5% Ringer's lactate solution) and increase the infusion rate until resolution of ketonuria. Continue to evaluate her blood glucose every 2 hours while the insulin drip is running (Table 5–5).

IX. **For a patient who is having an elective cesarean** and is admitted the morning of her surgery:

A. Document fetal lung maturity.
B. Verify that the patient has no evidence of an upper respiratory infection.
C. Obtain routine laboratory tests (CBC, FBS, urinalysis) and have 2 units of packed red blood cells typed and held.
D. Check the patient's chart for a signed consent for surgery (and for sterilization if desired).
E. Instruct the patient to be NPO after midnight, and to shower in the morning.
F. Instruct her to omit her bedtime and morning insulin.
G. Obtain a capillary glucose test upon arrival, before surgery as needed, and immediately after surgery. If her blood glu-

TABLE 5–5.
An Example of How a Continuous Insulin Infusion May Be Administered

Blood Glucose (mg/dL)	Insulin (units/hr)	Fluids (125 units/hr)
<100	0.5	D5LR
100–140	1.0	D5LR
141–180	1.5	NS
181–220	2.0	NS
>220	2.5	NS

D5LR = dextrose 5% Ringer's lactate solution; NS = normal saline.

cose is <80 mg/dL, infuse D5LR. If >120, administer insulin.

H. Upon admission, administer IV LR at 125 mL/hr.

I. Place a Foley catheter to gravity just before surgery.

J. Manage the patient's operation as a normal postoperative cesarean section, except for blood glucose and insulin dosage as detailed in the next section.

X. Immediate Postpartum Management

A. Most diabetic patients, especially those in Class A_2, will not require insulin for the first 24 hours after delivery. Insulin given at this time may trigger hypoglycemia.

B. The tight glycemic control needed antepartum to improve fetal outcome is loosened in the immediate postpartum period. Values of 150–200 mg/dL are acceptable.

C. Initially infuse LR. Examine the capillary glucose value immediately after delivery, again in 1–2 hours, and then before all meals and at bedtime (or every 4–6 hours in patients who are NPO). (Frequency may vary depending on the last dose of insulin.) Check the patient's urine for ketones at every void. If the patient becomes ketotic, replace LR with D5LR.

D. Have the nurse call you if the patient's blood glucose is <60 or >200 mg/dL. Test all urine samples for glucose and acetone, and have the nurse notify you of all urine glucose levels >2+, or ketone levels >1+.

1. If her urine glucose is ≥2+, check her capillary glucose. If the capillary plasma value is:
   a. <200 mg/dL, administer no insulin (some prefer not to give insulin if BS is ≤250 mg/dL)
   b. >200 mg/dL, administer insulin according to the following sliding scale:

201–250	2 units regular
251–300	4 units regular
301–350	6 units regular
>350	Notify house officer

2. Increase her insulin dosage if ketonuria is present.

E. In those patients who **do require** postpartum insulin while on an ADA diet, the morning dose should be approximately 20 units NPH, or half the prepregnancy insulin requirements. These guidelines are good empiric starting points.

F. The **ADA diet** is calculated as follows:

1. **During pregnancy: 30 kcal/kg actual body weight**
2. **After pregnancy: 30 kcal/kg ideal body weight (up to 2,600 calories)**
3. Calculate patient's ideal body weight according to the formula:
   a. $45.5 + [2.3 \times (\text{height in inches} - 60)] = \text{kilograms}$.
   b. For example:
      $45.5 + [2.3 \times (67 - 60)] = 61.6$ kg (135.5 pounds).
4. If your patient is breast feeding, an extra 500 kcal may be added to the calculated value.

XI. Special Discharge Orders

A. **Class A.** Schedule a FBS or a 3-hour glucose tolerance test (GTT) to be performed just before your patient's 6-week follow-up visit. If test results are abnormal, refer her to an internist (or diabetologist). Advise and plan weight reduction.

B. **Class A_2.** If diabetes has resolved after delivery, schedule a FBS or 3-hour GTT for your patient in 6 weeks and arrange an appointment with an internist. If her diabetic condition persists after delivery, schedule the internal medicine appointment within 1 week for evaluation and follow-up.

C. Refer patients who were on a regimen of insulin therapy before pregnancy to their diabetologist within 1–2 weeks after delivery. Do not order a GTT.

D. Send all patients who are not on a regimen of insulin therapy home with urine glucose strips. Instruct them to check their morning urine for sugar every 1–2 days, and if glucosuria develops to notify you immediately. Have these patients promptly evaluated for diabetes.

BIBLIOGRAPHY

American College of Obstetricians and Gynecologists: *Management of Diabetes Mellitus in Pregnancy*. Technical Bulletin No. 92, 1986.

Drury MI, Stronge JM, Foley ME, et al: Pregnancy in the diabetic patient: Timing and mode of delivery. *Obstet Gynecol* 1983; 62:279–282.

Gabbe SG: Management of diabetes mellitus in pregnancy. *Am J Obstet Gynecol* 1985; 153:824–828.

Janovic L, Peterson CM: Screening for gestational diabetes, optimum timing and criteria for retesting. *Diabetes* 1985; 34(suppl 2):21–23.

Mills JL, Simpson JL, Driscoll SG, et al: Incidence of spontaneous abortion among normal women and insulin-dependent diabetic women whose pregnancies were identified within 21 days of conception. *N Engl J Med* 1988; 319:1617–1623.

Pedersen J, Pedersen LM, Anderson B: Assessors of fetal perinatal mortality in diabetic pregnancy: Analysis of 1,332 pregnancies in the Copenhagen series 1946–1972. *Diabetes* 1974; 23:302–305.

White P: Diabetes mellitus in pregnancy. *Clin Perinatol* 1974; 1:331–347.

Yeast JD, Porreco RP, Ginsberg HN: The use of continuous insulin infusion for the peripartum management of pregnant diabetic women. *Am J Obstet Gynecol* 1978; 131:861.

HEPATITIS* 6

I. General Information for All Types of Viral Hepatitis

A. Background

1. **Definition.** The term *hepatitis* refers to liver inflammation.
2. **Viral hepatitis** is the most common cause of jaundice in pregnancy.

B. Prevention of Disease in Health Care Providers

1. Wear gloves and protective covering when the potential for coming into contact with the patient's blood, excreta, and body secretions is present.
2. All patients and their specimens are to be regarded as infected and the disease considered contagious.

II. Hepatitis A Virus (HAV)

A. Background (Table 6–1)

1. **Etiology.** HAV is caused by a 27 nm RNA virus.
2. **Incidence.** Approximately 34,200 new cases occur each year in the United States general population.
3. **Transmission** is usually fecal-oral (Table 6–2).
4. The **incubation** period ranges between 15 and 50 days, with a mean of 30. The virus is shed into the feces about 2 weeks before symptoms appear, persists for 1–2 weeks after the onset of clinical illness, and is absent after the patient develops jaundice. No carrier state exists. Long-term immunity follows recovery.
5. **Perinatal Morbidity and Mortality.** HAV is associated with prematurity and an increased spontaneous abortion rate.
6. **Maternal Morbidity and Mortality.** Maternal mortality occurs at a rate of 0.6%. HAV only rarely progresses to

*The author would like to acknowledge the valuable assistance of Ted Bader, M.D, in the preparation of this chapter.

TABLE 6–1.

Types of Viral Hepatitis

Infectious Agent	Hepatitis A	Hepatitis B	Hepatitis C
Causative agent	RNA virus (27 nm)	DNA virus (42 nm)	RNA virus (30–60 nm)
Transmission	Fecal-oral	Parenteral or body fluids	Parenteral or body fluids
Incubation period	15–50 days	45–160 days	18–100 days
Time of maximum infectivity	Prodrome	Prodrome (HB carrier: anytime)	Prodrome
Diagnosis	HA antibody (IgM and IgG)	HBsAg HBcAb HBsAb HBeAg (HB carrier: HBsAg)	HCAb
Carrier state	None	5%–10% become carriers	50%
Chronic forms	None	Chronic active hepatitis	Chronic active hepatitis

TABLE 6–2.
Vertical Transmission of Hepatitis

		Hepatitis B		
Infectious Agent	Hepatitis A	Active	Carrier	Hepatitis C
Transmission risk to infant	Low	1st and 2nd trim: $<10\%$ 3rd trim: 65%	HBeAg present: 75%–95% HBeAg absent: $<5\%$ HBcAg present: $<5\%$	Unknown
Newborn disease	Rare—would manifest at 14–30 days of life	Manifests at 30–120 days; disease is mild, rarely severe	Manifests at 30–120 days; disease may be fatal	
Infant complications	None	Carrier state common	Carrier state is common; 10–20 years later cirrhosis or hepatoma may develop	

fulminant hepatitis. No evidence exists to implicate HAV in progressing to chronic liver disease.

B. Evaluation

1. **History.** Patients often have a 2 to 5 day prodrome of mild fever, generalized malaise, myalgias, fatigue, weakness, anorexia, nausea and vomiting, and abdominal pain. After the prodrome, the icteric phase (icteric sclera, jaundice, light-colored stools, dark urine) occurs. This may be accompanied by increased anorexia, extreme fatigue, and mild pruritus. Symptoms last 10–15 days, followed by a gradual recovery. Rarely, fulminant hepatitis may occur (1/1,000 cases).
2. **Diagnostic Data** (Fig 6–1)
   a. The presence of IgM (immunoglobulin gamma M) antibody to hepatitis A is diagnostic of a current HAV infection and is usually present at the onset of jaundice.
   b. In a typical case, aspartate aminotransferase (ASP; SGOT) may rise to 1,000, and the alanine aminotransferase (ALT; SGPT) may rise to 2,000.

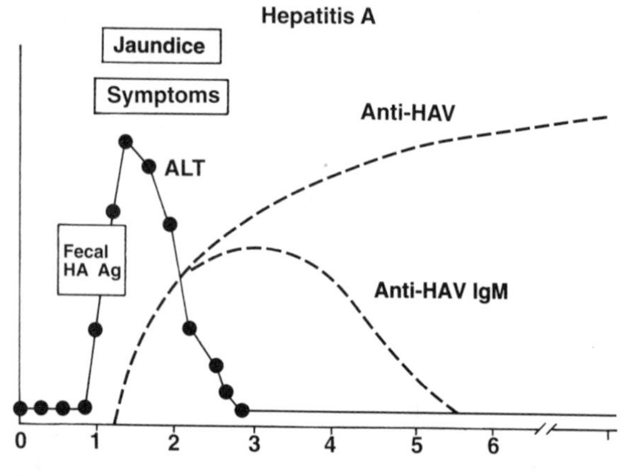

FIG 6–1.
Clinical, serologic, and biochemical course of typical type A hepatitis. *HA Ag* = hepatitis A antigen; *ALT* = alanine aminotransferase; *Anti-HAV* = antibody to hepatitis A virus.

c. In some cases a cholestatic picture occurs, with an elevated alkaline phosphatase and bilirubin accompanied by marked pruritus and light stools.
d. Infrequently the patient may become hypoalbuminemic, hypoglycemic, and may develop a coagulopathy.
e. IgG antibody to HAV persists after the infection has resolved. IgM antibody may last 4 to 6 months.

C. Therapeutic Management

1. Pregnancy does not alter management. Treatment supports the goal of **adequate nutrition.** In severe cases parenteral nutrition may be required. **Avoid hepatotoxic drugs** and drugs requiring liver metabolism.
2. **Immunoglobulin G** (IgG) should be given to all contacts without serologic documentation of infection (to facilitate rapid administration and to decrease the overall cost of care).
   a. IgG may be administered prophylactically (0.02 ml/kg body weight) if given within 2 weeks of exposure.
   b. IgG is a sterilized pooled serum solution unable to transmit infection (including human immunodeficiency virus).
   c. IgG is 80%–90% effective in preventing or modifying the course of illness.

III. Hepatitis B Virus (HBV)

A. Background

1. **Etiology.** HBV is caused by a 42 nm DNA virus.
2. **Incidence.** Approximately 22,800 reported new cases develop each year in the United States general population. It is believed that this infection is under reported and as many as 300,000 cases per year may actually occur.
3. **Transmission** is by contact with blood or semen. This includes percutaneous transmission in intravenous drug abusers, health care workers with accidental percutaneous exposure, maternal-neonatal vertical transmission, and sexual promiscuity of affected individuals.
4. **Incubation** ranges from 45–160 days, with a mean of 60–120 days.
5. **Perinatal Morbidity and Mortality.** It is thought by most viral hepatitis experts that significant in utero infection of the fetus by the hepatitis B virus does not occur. This is because administration of hepatitis B immune

globulin (HBIG) at birth dramatically reduces perinatal infection. (HBIG does not work if the infection has occurred more than 7 days previously.) The serological findings of chronic infection in the newborn probably reflect contamination from the mother's blood.

6. **Maternal Morbidity and Mortality**
   a. The maternal mortality rate is the same as that experienced in the nonpregnant patient.
   b. A **carrier state** may develop. A carrier is defined as a person who is HBsAg positive on two occasions at least 6 months apart. In the United States the carrier rate is 0.1%–0.5% (as high as 50% of adults in endemic areas). The resolution rate of chronic carriers is 1% per year.
   c. Twenty-five percent of HBV carriers develop chronic active hepatitis. Pregnancy does not increase the propensity of a patient to develop fulminant hepatitis.
   d. Fulminant hepatitis associated with deep coma has an 80% mortality rate.
7. **Screening.** The Centers for Disease Control and the American College of Obstetricians and Gynecologists recommend that **all pregnant women** be screened for hepatitis B surface antigen (HbsAg). The following **high-risk groups** account for only 50% of carrier women.
   a. Women of Asian, Pacific Islands, or Alaskan Eskimo descent, whether immigrant or US born
   b. Women born in Haiti or sub-Sahara Africa
   c. Women with histories of:
      1) Work in a health care or public safety field*
      2) Acute or chronic liver disease
      3) Work or treatment in a hemodialysis unit*
      4) Work or residence in an institution for the mentally retarded
      5) Rejection as a blood donor
      6) Repeated blood transfusions, as in sickle cell disease, thalassemia
      7) Frequent occupational exposure to blood in medical-dental settings (dental hygienist, nurse, physician)*
      8) Household contact with HBV carrier or hemodialysis patient*

*Denotes patients at highest risk.

9) Multiple episodes of venereal diseases (prostitutes)
10) Percutaneous use of illicit drugs

d. Women at risk for acquired immunodeficiency syndrome

B. Evaluation

1. **Clinical.** The typical features of hepatitis detailed under HAV (Part II) occur in the majority of patients; however, the prodrome in HBV usually lasts 2–4 weeks. A prodrome of arthralgia, arthritis, rash, angioedema, and, rarely, hematuria and proteinuria may occur in 5% to 10% of patients. Infrequently one may develop fulminant hepatitis with encephalopathy or coma (1/100 patients with HBV, versus 1/1,000 with HAV).
2. **Diagnostic Data** (Fig 6–2)
   a. Many serologic antigen markers exist for **HBV** (Table 6–3), but the three most important are hepatitis B surface antigen **(HBsAg),** hepatitis B core antigen (HBcAg), and hepatitis B envelope antigen (**HBeAg;** also known as soluble antigen).
   b. **HBsAg** appears in the blood approximately 6 weeks after hepatitis exposure (2 weeks before clinical symptoms are present) and persists for about 3 months (1–2 weeks after symptoms resolve).
   c. About the time that HBsAg disappears, **HBsAb** can be detected.
   d. **HBeAg** correlates with HBV replication, and is a sign of high infectivity. It is only transiently present and occurs early in the infection.
   e. **HBcAb** is present during the "window" phase, when HBsAg has cleared and the HBsAb has not appeared.

C. Management

1. As with HAV, management is supportive.
2. In the event of hepatic encephalopathy
   a. Dietary protein should be restricted and
   b. **Lactulose syrup** administered in a 50 mL dose (65 g/dL) every 2 hours until diarrhea occurs. (It takes 24–48 hours to see the response to lactulose.) The dose may then be adjusted so that the patient has two to four loose stools daily.
   c. Alternatively, or in addition to the lactulose, **neomycin,** 0.5 g every 6 hours, should be administered orally.

TABLE 6–3.

Hepatitis Nomenclature*

Viral Type	Terminology	Comments
Hepatitis A		
HAV	Hepatitis A virus	Etiologic agent of "infectious" hepatitis, a picornavirus: single serotype
Anti-HAV	Antibody to HAV	Detectable onset of symptoms, lifetime persistence
IgM anti-HAV	IgM class antibody to HAV	Indicates recent infection with hepatitis A: positive up to 4–6 months after infection
Hepatitis B		
HBV	Hepatitis B virus	Etiologic agent of "serum" or "long-incubation" hepatitis; also known as Dane particle
HBsAg	Hepatitis B surface antigen	Surface antigen(s) of HBV detectable in large quantity in serum: several subtypes identified
HBeAg	Hepatitis B e antigen	Soluble antigen: correlates with HBV replication, high titer HBV in serum, and infectivity of serum
HBcAg	Hepatitis B core antigen	No commercial test available; present only in the liver, not serum
Anti-HBs (HBsAb)	Antibody to HBsAg	Indicates past infection with and immunity to HBV, passive antibody from HBIG, or immune response from HBV vaccine
Anti-HBe (HBeAb)	Antibody to HBeAg	Presence in serum of HBsAg carrier suggests low titer of HBV
Anti-HBc (HBcAb)	Antibody to HBcAg	Indicates past infection with HBV at some undefined time
IGM anti-HBc	IgM class antibody to HBcAg	Indicates recent infection with HBV; positive for 4–6 months after infection

Delta hepatitis		
δ virus	Delta virus	Etiologic agent of delta hepatitis; may only cause infection in presence of HBV
δ-Ag	Delta antigen	Indicates past or present infection with delta virus (the Delta antigen assay is not available commercially)
Anti-δ	Antibody to delta antigen	
Hepatitis C		
HCV	Hepatitis C virus	Causes at least 85% of non-A non-B (NANB) hepatitis; the remaining cases on NANB hepatitis are a diagnosis of exclusion: epidemiology parallels that of hepatitis
Anti HC	Antibody to HCV	The antibody is detected 3–4 months after an acute infection
Hepatitis E	Epidemic non-A, non-B hepatitis	Causes large epidemics in Asia, North Africa; fecal-oral or waterborne
Immune globulins		
IG	Immune globulin (previously ISG [immune serum globulin], or gamma globulin)	Contains antibodies to HAV, low-titer antibodies to HBV
HBIG	Hepatitis B immune globulin	Contains a high titer of antibodies to HBV

*From Immunization Practices Advisory Committee Recommendations for Protection Against Viral Hepatitis. *MMWR* 1985; 34:313–335, June 7, 1985. Used by permission.

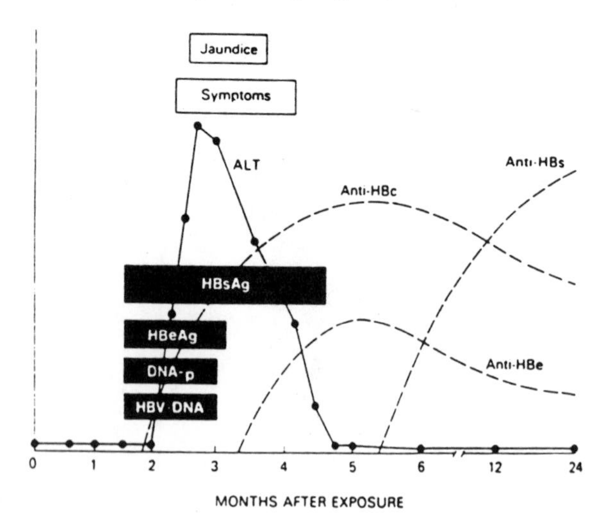

FIG 6–2.
Clinical and serologic course of a typical case of acute type B hepatitis. *HBsAg* = hepatitis B surface antigen; *HBeAg* = hepatitis B e antigen; *DNA-p* = DNA polymerase; *HBV-DNA* = hepatitis B virus DNA; *ALT* = alanine aminotransferase; *anti-HBc* = antibody to hepatitis B core antigen; *anti-HBe* = antibody to hepatitis B e antigen; *anti-HBs* = antibody to hepatitis B surface antigen. (From Mandell G, Douglas R, Bennett J: *Principles and Practice of Infectious Diseases*. New York, John Wiley & Sons, 1985. Used by permission.)

d. Consider transferring the patient to a liver transplant center for observation.

D. Effect on Pregnancy

1. The fetus may become infected more frequently from the viremia if the virus develops during pregnancy than in a mother who is chronically HBsAg positive.
2. More than 90% of maternal-fetal transmissions occur at delivery. Cesarean section does not reduce this risk.
3. Neonatal prophylaxis is mandatory for all infants born to HBsAg positive mothers.

E. Prevention of Disease in the Neonate

1. The neonate of any mother who is HBsAg positive should be immunized, both passively with hepatitis B immunoglobulin (HBIG) and actively with a hepatitis B vaccine at birth. The status of the mother with respect to the HBeAg is not relevant to the decision to immunize the neonate, although if HBeAg is present it is predictive of a higher transmission rate from mother to infant.
2. **Procedure for Neonatal Immunization**
   a. Wash the anterior aspect of the thighs of the neonate so that maternal blood is not inoculated with the needle stick.
   b. Administer **HBIG** (0.5 ml) IM in the anterior aspect of one thigh and **HB vaccine** (0.5 ml) IM in the opposite thigh within 48 hours after birth. (This is the ideal method; however, HBIG may be given up to 7 days after birth, and HB vaccine may be administered at any time.)
   c. Repeat the HB vaccine at 1 and 6 months.
   d. Test the infant for HBsAg and anti-HBsAg at 12 to 15 months of age.

IV. Hepatitis C (HCV; Formerly Non-A Non-B Hepatitis)

A. Background

1. **Incidence.** Approximately 2,400 new cases develop each year in the United States general population. As with HBV, this reported figure is thought to underestimate the true incidence of HCV.
2. **Etiology.** The information on non-A non-B hepatitis (NANBH) is currently in flux. As of the time of this writing, hepatitis C virus (HCV) is thought to cause at least 85% of NANB cases. Hepatitis C is caused by an RNA virus, between 30–60nm in size. The remaining cases of NANBH also may be caused by HCV (but our assays may not be sensitive enough to detect these cases), or by a second virus not yet identified.
3. **Transmission** is percutaneous. Since all blood is screened for HBcAb and HBsAg, HCV has become the most frequent form of hepatitis occurring after blood transfusion. If the liver function tests of the donated blood show elevated values, HCV is presumed present and the blood is discarded.
4. The **incubation period** is 18–100 days.

5. **Evaluation.** The clinical illness is similar to that of HBV. Hepatitis C may be detected by an assay for hepatitis C antibody (HCAb) (Fig 6–3). The antibody is not detected in blood until 3 to 4 months after the acute episode. In the right clinical setting, when the HCAb assay is negative, elevated liver enzymes may be suggestive of its presence.
6. **Therapeutic Management.** As with HAV and HBV, management is supportive. The American College of Obstetricians and Gynecologists recommends treatment with IG 0.06 ml/kg after exposure to HCV (the efficacy of this is unproven, as compared with hepatitis A where it is well proven). This infection is not well studied in pregnancy.

V. Hepatitis E (Formerly Called Epidemic Non-A, Non-B Hepatitis)

A. Background. A 32nm RNA virus which has caused large outbreaks of acute non-A, non-B Hepatitis in Southeast Asia, India, Africa and Mexico. It is transmitted by fecal-oral means

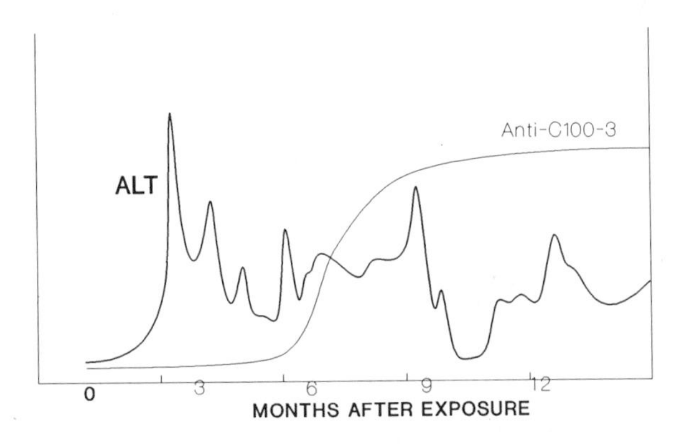

FIG 6–3.
Graph demonstrates that the rise and fall of this biochemical marker is unrelated to disease activity and clinical infectivity. ALT = alanine aminotransferase; Anti-C100-3 = the Standard Anti-C antibody. (Courtesy of Dr. Ted Bader.)

and thus is different from Hepatitis C (percutaneous non-A, non-B Hepatitis).

B. Clinical presentation. Hepatitis E is an acute, self-limited disease which is very similar to the other enterically transmitted hepatitis, HAV. The outcome is usually benign but with the peculiar feature that pregnant women have had from 20% to 100% case-mortality rate in epidemics. The primary time of fatality has been in the third trimester.

C. Diagnosis. No serological tests are available. Hepatitis E can be suspected if the patient has a travel history in the past 3 months and a clinical picture of Hepatitis A but who tests negative for IgM-HAV. A stool specimen can be sent to the Center for Disease Control (CDC) for confirmation.

D. Implications. There have been no **de novo** cases of Hepatitis E arising in the United States. There have been a number of imported cases, principally from Mexico. While the CDC has not issued a formal statement, it seems prudent to advise pregnant women not to travel to Southeast Asia, India, Africa or rural Mexico, particularly during their third trimester.

E. Treatment. There is no evidence that United States manufactured immune globulin will prevent Hepatitis E. The best means for avoiding it are to avoid contaminated food or water.

VI. Hepatitis D (Delta Agent)

A. Background

1. **Etiology.** An RNA virus (or portion of a virus) that requires the presence of HBV for infectivity.
2. **Incidence.** The exact incidence is unknown, but it is less than that of HBV. In the United States intravenous drug abusers are the principle group at risk. Homosexuals in the United States have not yet acquired the Delta agent.
3. **Transmission, incubation, and evaluation** are all the same as for HBV. Commercialized screening for the delta antibody is available. Presence of the Delta antibody means that the patient is currently infected. This test should be ordered only if the patient is HBsAg positive (since the Delta virus uses HBsAg as its outer coat). Vertical transmission from mother to infant is of minor epidemiologic relevance, and thus routine screening of patients positive for HBsAg is not recommended. If a patient is known to be positive for the delta antibody, the recommendations for **management of**

the neonate are the same as those for neonates positive for HBsAg alone.

BIBLIOGRAPHY

Alter JJ: The hepatitis C virus and its relationship to the clinical spectrum of NANB hepatitis, in *Common Liver Problems: An Update on Practice and Science*. Chicago, The American Association for the Study of Liver Diseases, 1990; pp 287–303.

American College of Obstetricians and Gynecologists: *Guidelines for Hepatitis B Virus Screening and Vaccination During Pregnancy*. Committee Opinion No. 78, January 1990.

Immunization Practices Advisory Committee. Recommendations for protection against viral hepatitis. *MMWR* 1985; 34:313–335.

Krawcznski K: Epidemic non-A, non-B hepatitis, in *New Frontiers in Liver Disease*. Chicago, The American Association for the Study of Liver Diseases, 1989; pp 151–169.

Progress in chronic disease prevention. *MMWR* 1989; 38:507, July 28.

Rustgi VK, Cooper JN: *Gastrointestinal and Hepatic Complications in Pregnancy*. New York, John Wiley & Sons.

Summers PR, Bean B, Gray BJ: Hepatitis B in obstetrics and gynecology. *Obstet Gynecol Forum* 1988; 2(2).

Zanetti AR, Ferroni P, Magliano EM, et al: Perinatal transmission of the hepatitis B virus and the HBV-associated delta agent from mothers to offspring in northern Italy. *J Med Virol* 1982; 9L:139–148.

CHRONIC HYPERTENSION 7

I. Background

A. Definition. BP >140/90 mm Hg on two occasions more than 6 hours apart, before pregnancy (Fig 7–1 and Table 7–1).

B. Incidence. Chronic hypertension (HTN) is present in 2% of pregnancies.

C. Etiology

1. The cause of chronic HTN is detailed in Table 7–2.
2. Primary essential HTN accounts for most chronic HTN seen during pregnancy. An intensive workup of HTN need not be performed during pregnancy, but a thorough physical examination must be performed and consultation with an internist must be obtained if concern arises regarding the possibility of secondary HTN.

D. Perinatal Morbidity and Mortality. Intrauterine growth retardation (IUGR) is increased in infants born to mothers with HTN. The perinatal mortality rate is 8% to 15%.

E. Maternal Morbidity and Mortality

1. Thirty percent of patients with an elevated BP during pregnancy have essential HTN (not pregnancy-induced HTN).
2. Between 10% and 50% of patients with chronic HTN will develop superimposed pregnancy-induced HTN during their pregnancy.
3. These patients are at risk for abruptio placentae (incidence 0.45%–10% depending on the duration and severity of the HTN).

II. Evaluation

A. History. Inquire into:

1. A family history of HTN
2. Previous HTN treated with medications

TABLE 7–1.
Cardiovascular Changes in Pregnancy*

Parameter	Amount of Change	Timing
Arterial blood		
Pressures		
Systolic	↓ 4–6 mm HG	All bottom at 20–24 wk, then rise gradually to prepregnancy values at term
Diastolic	↓ 8–15 mm HG	
Mean†	↓ 6–10 mm HG	
Heart rate	↑ 12–18 bpm	Early 2nd trimester, then stable
Stroke volume	↑ 10%–30%	Early 2nd trimester, then stable
Cardiac output	↑ 33%–45%	Peaks in early 2nd trimester, then stable until term‡

*From Main DM, Main EK: *Obstetrics and Gynecology. A Pocket Reference.* St Louis, Mosby–Year Book, 1984. Used by permission.

†Mean arterial BP is calculated by the formula $MAP = \frac{S + 2D}{3}$.

A more manageable formula is $MAP = D + \frac{1}{3}(S - D)$.

‡The timing of the changes in cardiac output is controversial. Initial studies suggested a gradual rise to a peak at 26–28 wk with a fall as term approached. More recent studies indicate an earlier rise in output that remains stable until delivery. The difference may be related to techniques and maternal position.

TABLE 7–2.
Etiology of Chronic HTN

- Primary essential HTN
- Secondary HTN
  - Arterial
    - Coarctation of the aorta
    - Renal arterial stenosis
  - Chronic renal disease
  - Neurologic disorders
  - Endocrine disorders
    - Acromegaly
    - Cushing's syndrome
    - Conn's syndrome (primary hyperaldosteronism)
    - Pheochromocytoma
  - Drug-induced
    - Amphetamines
    - Cocaine

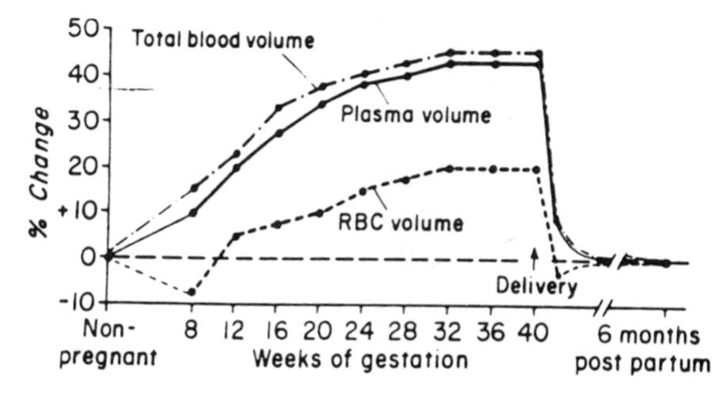

FIG 7–1.

Circulatory changes in pregnancy. Changes in blood volume, plasma volume, red cell volume, and cardiac output begin in the first trimester, rise most sharply in the second, and peak in the early third trimester. These curves were constructed from various reports in the literature and illustrate trends in percent change from nonpregnant values. It is important to realize that there can be large individual variation. For example, while it is accepted that the average maximum increase in blood volume is between 40% and 50%, individuals have had a reported increase in their volume as little as 20% and as much as 100%. Cardiac output remains elevated during the third trimester if measured in the lateral position. (From Bonica JJ: *Obstetric Analgesia and Anesthesia,* ed 2. Amsterdam, World Federation of Societies of Anesthesiologists, 1980, p 2. Used by permission.)

3. Current use of medications, particularly monoamine oxidase inhibitors
4. Monoamine oxidase inhibitor intolerance (HTN develops after ingesting foods containing tyramine or cold medications, which include such agents as phenylpropanolamine.)
5. History suggestive of a pheochromocytoma (frequent heart palpitations, excessive and inappropriate sweating, anxiety, facial pallor)
6. Frequent previous hospitalizations during pregnancy
7. Primary aldosteronism (Symptoms include polyuria, proximal muscle weakness, paresthesias, all of which are secondary to hypokalemia.)
8. Thyrotoxicosis (fatigue, palpitations, heat intolerance, weight loss, increased frequency of bowel movement)

9. History of systemic lupus erythematosus, diabetes mellitus, pyelonephritis, urinary tract disorders (may result in chronic nephritis)

B. **Physical Examination.** Perform a complete physical examination with specific attention directed to the following:

1. Examine the **eyes** for findings suggestive of hyperthyroidism. Look for periorbital swelling, exophthalmos chemosis, conjunctival infection, and proptosis. Perform **funduscopic** eye examination to evaluate for long-standing and accelerated HTN.
2. Palpate the **thyroid gland** for enlargement.
3. Measure the **BP** in her arms bilaterally with the appropriate size cuff and **listen for bruits. Palpate the femoral arteries** to exclude aortic coarctation.
4. Auscultate the **abdomen** (in early gestations) to rule out a murmur consistent with renal artery stenosis.
5. Examine the patient's **general appearance.** Truncal obesity, plethora, muscle wasting, virilization or hirsutism, and thin skin are suggestive of Cushing's syndrome.
6. Perform a clinical evaluation of the chest, as outlined in Table 7–3.

C. **Diagnostic Data**

1. The **laboratory evaluation** should include:
   a. **Urinalysis** to screen for renal disease
   b. **Hematocrit**
   c. Plasma **potassium** (Hypokalemia, if the patient is not on diuretics, is suggestive of early hyperaldosteronism; hyperkalemia may suggest renal parenchymal disease.)
   d. Plasma **creatinine** (if elevated is suggestive of renal parenchymal disease), **calcium,** and **uric acid** levels
   e. Fasting serum **cholesterol** and triglycerides
   f. **One hour postglucola** if not recently obtained (Glucose intolerance, if accompanied by truncal obesity, plethora, muscle wasting, virilization or hirsutism, and thin skin, is suggestive of Cushing's syndrome.)
   g. **EKG** (Left ventricular hypertrophy may suggest chronic HTN.)
   h. Consider obtaining a **24-hour urine** collection for protein and creatinine in the presence of severe HTN.
   i. Consider sending **liver enzymes** to provide a baseline evaluation of liver function in the event that the patient develops superimposed preeclampsia

TABLE 7–3.
Clinical Evaluation of the Chest*

A. Cardiac auscultation[1]
1. Sounds: First sound is louder with exaggerated splitting; second sound minimally changed; third sound is heard loudly in a majority of women; a fourth sound is heard only occasionally.
2. Murmurs: Early systolic ejection murmur (occasionally midsystolic) develops in greater than 90% of women; 18% were grade I and 82% were grade II. Some (18%) also had a soft diastolic "flow" murmur.

B. Chest x-ray
Diaphragm elevates (approximately 4 cm) with subsequent lateral and anterior displacement of the heart significantly changing the cardiac silhouette. Flaring of ribs is also noted with an increase in the subcostal angle from 68 degrees in early pregnancy to 103 degrees at term.

C. ECG[2]
A recent study of 102 women with serial ECGs through pregnancy and postpartum has better defined the normal range. There are no clinically significant changes in cardiac rhythm or in ECG intervals. The QRS amplitude increases slightly. On average there is a mild but significant left axis shift in both QRS and T-wave axis, particularly in the third trimester. However, there is great individual variation with a substantial minority exhibiting axis changes to the right (maximum changes were 40 degrees either direction). Other studies have noted the development of a Q wave in lead III and an increased frequency of ectopic beats (both PAC and PVC).

D. Echocardiogram[3]
Serial studies on normal gravidas found progressive left ventricular enlargement (approximately 10% increase in end-diastolic ventricular size). However, shortening characteristics including ejection fraction were not altered. Overall, despite increased heart rate and left ventricular size, ventricular function was well preserved.

Selected references:

1. Cutforth R, MacDonald CB: Heart sounds and murmurs in pregnancy, *Am Heart J.* 1966; 71:741.
2. Carruth JE et al: The electrocardiogram in normal pregnancy, *Am Heart J.* 1981; 102:1075.
3. Katz R, Karliner JS, Resnick R: Effects of a natural volume overload state (pregnancy) on left ventricular performance in normal human subjects, *Circulation* 1978; 58:434.

*From Main DM, Main EK: *Obstetrics and Gynecology. A Pocket Reference.* St Louis, Mosby–Year Book, 1984. Used by permission.

2. **Antenatal Surveillance**
   a. **Ultrasound Evaluation**
      1) Obtain a baseline scan at 16–18 weeks to confirm gestational age.
      2) Beginning at 26–28 weeks, obtain follow-up scans

every 3–4 weeks with serial measurements (to rule out IUGR).
3) If preeclampsia develops, begin serial scans at the time of diagnosis (if before 26–28 weeks).

b. **Antepartum Testing** (Please refer to Appendix L.)
1) Begin at 32–34 weeks in patients with uncomplicated HTN.
2) Begin at the time of diagnosis of superimposed preeclampsia or IUGR.
3) If the patient's dates are poor, consider amniocentesis at 38–39 weeks to evaluate fetal lung maturity for possible delivery.

III. Therapeutic Management

A. Outpatient Management

1. Patients with chronic HTN should continue on the same medications they were taking before conception, with the exception of diuretics and angiotensin-converting enzyme inhibitors (i.e., Captopril).
2. **Atenolol** (Tenormin), a β-selective adrenoreceptor blocking agent, is the newest drug of choice. Dosing is usually 50–100 mg/day orally, and may be increased up to 250 mg daily.
3. Previously, **methyldopa** (Aldomet), whose metabolite stimulates central α-adrenergic receptors, was the drug of choice. It is administered in 250–500 mg doses orally every 6 hours. It is still frequently used.
4. **Labetalol** (Normodyne; Trandate) is a combination α-blocker and β-blocker that can easily be started during pregnancy. The dose is 100 mg orally every 6–8 hours to a maximum of 800 mg in 24 hours.
5. If the patient's BP decreases markedly during the first or early second trimester, consider lowering the dosage or discontinuing her anti-HTN medication. When BP elevations are noted after 20 weeks, promptly evaluate the patient for superimposed preeclampsia. In the absence of preeclampsia, consider reinitiating antihypertensive therapy (especially in the presence of diastolic BP >100) versus continued observation until delivery. Base the decision on the severity of the patient's HTN.
6. The frequency of office visits correlates with disease severity. Initially, mildly hypertensive patients may be seen

as often as patients with uncomplicated pregnancies. Reevaluate the frequency of visits if the patient develops proteinuria or a sudden rise in **BP.** If either proteinuria or BP is severe, evaluate her in the labor and delivery unit.

7. Have the patient monitor her BP at least twice daily.

B. Inpatient Management

1. Patients who have been admitted for worsening HTN or superimposed preeclampsia are usually hospitalized for the duration of their pregnancies.
   a. If the gestation is near or at term, deliver the infant. Induce labor if the patient is not in labor and neither a fetal nor maternal indication exists to warrant a cesarean section.
   b. If the patient's condition is severe, consider immediate delivery regardless of gestational age. Induce if no indication for cesarean is present.
      1) Refer to Chapter 16 for management of patients with severe preeclampsia.
      2) In a **hypertensive emergency:**
         a) Administer **hydralazine.** The usual dose is 2.5 mg slow intravenous push. This may be repeated in 5 to 10 minutes if her BP does not decrease. Hydralazine requires 20 minutes for its full effect to be manifested. Aim for a diastolic BP ≥90 mm Hg. If the diastolic BP drops to less than 90 mm Hg, uteroplacental insufficiency may occur. The dosage may be increased as needed.
         b) Place a Foley **catheter** for strict monitoring of intake and output. **Central monitoring** may be necessary. Refer to Chapter 16, Tables 16-1 and 16-2, for indications and normal values of hemodynamic monitoring in pregnancy.
      3) **Monitor the fetus** carefully.
2. Patients in stable condition with gestations remote from term are managed similarly to patients with pregnancy-induced HTN receiving long-term antepartum care (see Chapter 16). Obtain an EKG and an ophthalmic examination.
3. If the patient is discharged home antepartum:
   a. Instruct her on the use of the BP cuff. Recommend that she purchase a cuff, record her BP every 4 hours dur-

ing the day, and bring the record to each office visit.

b. These patients are at an increased risk for placental abruption; thus, any vaginal bleeding should be promptly evaluated. Instruct your patient to report any bleeding occurrence to you immediately.

BIBLIOGRAPHY

Cunningham FG, Pritchard JA: How should hypertension during pregnancy be managed? *Med Clin North Am* 1984; 68:505.

Ferris TF: How should hypertension during pregnancy be managed? An internist's approach. *Med Clin North Am* 1984; 68:491.

Mishell DR, Brenner PF: *Management of Common Problems in Obstetrics and Gynecology*. Oradell, NJ, Medical Economics, 1988.

Sullivan JM: The hypertensive diseases of pregnancy and their management. *Adv Intern Med* 1982; 27:407.

CHRONIC IMMUNOLOGIC THROMBOCYTOPENIA 8

I. Background

A. **Chronic immunologic thrombocytopenia (ITP)** is the antibody-mediated destruction of maternal platelets. This condition may be diagnosed antenatally or it may be detected by means of a prenatal screening CBC in asymptomatic individuals. It is classified as follows:

1. Patients with an antenatal diagnosis of **ITP**
   a. **Intermediate ITP:** 50,000–100,000 platelets/mm^3
   b. **Severe ITP:** <50,000 platelets/mm^3
2. **Gestational** (incidental) **ITP:** Maternal platelet count <100,000 platelets per mm^3

B. **Incidence.** ITP primarily affects women in their reproductive years. It is the most common autoimmune disease of pregnancy, occurring in 0.01%–0.02% of pregnancies.

C. **Perinatal Morbidity and Mortality**

1. Up to 70% of all infants born to mothers with ITP have neonatal thrombocytopenia. Of infants at high risk for neonatal thrombocytopenia, 20%–26% have severe thrombocytopenia.
2. The perinatal mortality rate is 6%–14%, with deaths usually associated with prematurity, intracranial hemorrhage, and shock.

D. **Maternal Morbidity and Mortality.** The maternal mortality rate is 5.5% and maternal morbidity from hemorrhage (bleeding requiring transfusion) is 5%–26%.

E. **Etiology.** Immunoglobin G (IgG) (predominantly IgG_1, although frequently associated with IgG_3) directed against maternal platelets binds the platelets, causing them to be cleared by the reticuloendothelial system. IgG crosses the placenta and may precipitate fetal thrombocytopenia. The instigating factor for the antiplatelet antibody is unknown.

F. **Differential Diagnosis.** Before making the diagnosis of **ITP,** rule out:
   1. The use of medications (quinidine, sulfonamides, heparin, furosemide, and aspirin), which may cause thrombocytopenia
   2. Disseminated intravascular coagulation
   3. Lymphoproliferative disorders (Hodgkin's disease, leukemia, aplastic anemia)
   4. Systemic lupus erythematosus
   5. Hypersplenism
   6. Viral or bacterial infections (especially mononucleosis)
   7. Thrombotic thrombocytopenic purpura
   8. Hemolytic uremic syndrome
   9. Thyroid disease
   10. Sarcoidosis
   11. Preeclampsia

II. Evaluation

A. **History.** In an asymptomatic individual with newly detected **ITP,** elicit instigating factors of thrombocytopenia (preceding section). Question the patient about her bleeding tendency (antenatal menorrhagia, epistaxis, episodes of gastrointestinal (GI) bleeding, known retinal hemorrhages, joint bleeding, episodes of hematuria). Inquire whether she has noticed petechial or purpuric lesions, or subconjunctival hemorrhage.

B. **Physical Examination.** Perform a thorough physical examination. In patients with **ITP,** the skin may demonstrate petechial and purpuric lesions. During the ocular examination observe for subconjunctival hemorrhage and retinal hemorrhage (rare). Inspect her gums for bleeding. The remainder of the physical examination is usually within normal limits for pregnancy. Hypertension suggests preeclampsia, while splenomegaly and lymphadenopathy suggest infection (particularly mononucleosis), sarcoidosis, systemic lupus erythematosus, or a lymphoproliferative disorder.

C. **Diagnostic Data.** Evaluate the results of a CBC with differential and platelet count, platelet-associated IgG (antiplatelet antibody), antinuclear antibody titer, lupus anticoagulant, anticardiolipin, blood cultures, coagulation screen (usually prothrombin time), thyroid function tests, fibrinogen, VDRL, serum protein electrophoresis, and a bone marrow aspirate.

III. Therapeutic Management

A. Antepartum Management

1. Patients with thrombocytopenia (<100,000 platelets/mm^3) are admitted to the hospital when symptoms occur or when the platelet count is of concern to the admitting physician. **Less than 20,000 platelets/mm^3 mandates admission.**
2. Consult a **hematologist** regarding a diagnostic bone marrow biopsy and steroid therapy. **Initiate medical treatment according to the patient's clinical status when her platelet count drops below 50,000.**
   a. **Corticosteroids** are the primary treatment modality.
      1) Administer doses up to **60–100 mg/day of prednisone,** or 1.0 to 1.5 mg/kg/day (higher doses for platelet counts <10,000) until a response is evident. Divided dosages appear to be more effective than single daily doses or alternate-day therapy.
      2) A positive response is evidenced by a rise in the platelet count within 3 weeks and a decreasing incidence of new skin lesions.
      3) Gradually **taper the dose after a favorable response.** In those patients not responding within 3 weeks, consider another mode of therapy.
      4) Steroids decrease antiplatelet antibody production, interfere with antiplatelet antibody interaction with the platelet surface (thus increasing the amount of circulating, unbound antiplatelet antibody), decrease clearance of platelets coated with antiplatelet antibody, and improve abnormal capillary fragility.
      5) The circulating antibody concentration correlates inversely with the fetal platelet count; thus corticosteroids increase the risk of fetal thrombocytopenia.
      6) Additional **side effects** include maternal Cush-

ing's syndrome, psychosis, preeclampsia, fetal adrenal insufficiency, and growth retardation.

b. **Splenectomy** is indicated in patients who do not respond to corticosteroids, who have a life-threatening hemorrhage, or who are noncompliant.
   1) A favorable response is usually noted within a few hours after surgery; the optimal response occurs 1–3 weeks later.
   2) When the **platelet count rises above 1,000,000/mm^3,** acetylsalicylic acid (or a similar product) is recommended to prevent thromboembolism.
c. **Platelet transfusion** may be a temporary lifesaving measure in the presence of hemorrhage. Transfused platelets are destroyed rapidly by antiplatelet antibodies.
d. **Immunosuppressive drugs** (azathioprine, cyclophosphamide, and the vinca alkaloids) have been administered to patients who do not respond to corticosteroid therapy and splenectomy; however, these medications pose risks to the fetus of intrauterine growth retardation, teratogenicity, and oncogenicity, in addition to adverse maternal side effects. Their use remains experimental.
e. **Plasmapheresis** to remove antiplatelet antibodies may be used as an adjunct to primary treatment, or in an emergency when a rapid response is needed.
f. High-dose **intravenous immune globulin** (IV IgG) (400 mg/kg daily for 5 days) may transiently increase the platelet count. (IV IgG may interfere with the phagocyte Fc receptor–mediated immune clearance, thus allowing an increased number of platelets to circulate in the patient.)
   1) This therapy is not well documented in pregnancy, and IgG is thought to take up to 3 weeks to cross the placenta and positively affect fetal outcome.
   2) It is hypothesized that IV IgG also blocks the placental Fc receptors for transfer of the antiplatelet antibodies, thus reducing the amount of antibody transferred to the fetus.

3. After the diagnosis and therapeutic regimen are established, and the patient is stable, she may be discharged

home. Stress the importance of follow-up platelet counts, avoidance of injections or trauma, and avoidance of certain drugs (aspirin and nonsteroidal anti-inflammatory drugs unless otherwise indicated) to reduce the risk of bleeding.

B. Intrapartum Management

1. Patients in labor are usually **not** transfused before, during, or after delivery (unless symptomatic).
2. Each unit of platelets is from one donor, representing a **hepatitis C** risk of 3% and an acquired immunodeficiency syndrome risk of 1/100,000. Each unit will raise the platelet count by about 10,000 in a normal individual; however, in the **ITP** patient, the rise may be much less due to immune destruction of the transfused platelets.
3. Steroid and IV IgG therapy for patients in active labor with **ITP** is somewhat controversial. **Corticosteroids** are usually the primary therapy for patients in active labor.
   a. Proponents state that steroids decrease the incidence and severity of fetal thrombocytopenia.
   b. Opponents state that the opposite effect occurs (See Sections IIIA2a(4) and IIIA2a(5). In patients who continue to bleed despite steroid therapy, IV IgG may be administered.
4. **IV IgG** is transported inconsistently and unpredictably across the placenta. Some studies have suggested that the use of high-dose gamma globulin is safer and more effective than steroids in the treatment of maternal and fetal thrombocytopenia, but experience in pregnancy is limited at this point.

C. Delivery Management

1. A maternal platelet count ≥50,000 at delivery is preferable. Patients with lower counts, especially **<30,000, are at high risk for postpartum bleeding complications.** The primary risk of bleeding occurs with lacerations and incisions. **ITP rarely** causes postpartum uterine hemorrhage. Patients with platelet counts <50,000 may be treated with either steroids or IV IgG.
2. If the patient is taking steroids chronically, increase to stress doses (25 mg Solu-Medrol intravenous push or 100 mg Solu-Cortef intravenous push).
3. **Neonates with severe ITP may be predisposed to in-**

tracranial hemorrhage if delivered vaginally (with its inherent compression of the fetal cranium). It is important to identify neonates at high risk of thrombocytopenia and to examine their blood for evidence of severe **ITP.**

a. Mothers with **ITP diagnosed during the current pregnancy are at low risk** of having severe neonatal thrombocytopenia.
b. Mothers who carry an antenatal diagnosis of **ITP,** but who currently **do not have circulating antiplatelet antibodies,** are also at **low risk** of delivering a fetus with severe neonatal thrombocytopenia.
c. All patients other than those listed in C*1* and C2 are candidates for **evaluation of fetal platelet counts.** Two methods are available, both with inherent risks and benefits.
    1) **Percutaneous umbilical vein blood sampling**
        a) Technically this is the more difficult procedure; however, it is the more accurate of the two.
        b) Schedule the procedure to be performed before 38 weeks, because it cannot be performed intrapartum.
    2) **Fetal scalp blood sampling.** Drawbacks to the procedure include:
        a) The procedure may not be performed until the cervix is partially dilated and the membranes are ruptured. Intracranial hemorrhage may have occurred before the sampling, although this is considered to be infrequent.
        b) Significant bleeding may occur from the scalp lesion. (Firm pressure will usually prevent this.)
        c) If the specimen is contaminated with amniotic fluid, the platelet count may be artificially lowered.
        d) There is little time to do the procedure and get results.
        e) Clumping of platelets on the slide commonly occurs, giving erroneous results.
d. If a fetal platelet count cannot be determined antenatally in a patient at high risk for fetal thrombocytopenia, consider cesarean delivery.

D. Postpartum Management

1. The intensive medical care initiated antepartum must be continued through the initial postpartum period.
2. Breast milk may contain antiplatelet antibodies; however, these antibodies are destroyed in the infant's intestines and thus are not absorbed in their functional state. Corticosteroids may also be transmitted to the infant through the breast milk.

BIBLIOGRAPHY

Fehr J, Hofmann V, Kappeler U: Transient reversal of thrombocytopenia in idiopathic thrombocytopenia purpura by high-dose intravenous gama globulin. *N Engl J Med* 1982; 306:1254–1258.

Kelton JG, Inwood MJ, Barr RM, et al: The prenatal prediction of thrombocytopenia in infants of mothers with clinically diagnosed immune thrombocytopenia, *Am J Obstet Gynecol* 144:449–454.

Martin JN, Morrison JC, Files JC: Autoimmune thrombocytopenia purpura. Current concepts and recommended practices. *Am J Obstet Gynecol* 1984; 150:86–96.

Sacher RA: ITP in pregnancy and the newborn: Introduction. *Blut* 1989; 59:124–127.

Samuels P, Bussel JB, Braitman LE, et al: Estimation of the risk of thrombocytopenia in the offspring of pregnant women with presumed immune thrombocytopenic purpura. *N Engl J Med* 1990; 323:229–235.

Wordell JC: Immunotherapy of idiopathic thrombocytopenic purpura and autoimmune neutropenia. *Pharmacotherapy* 1987; 7:41S–47S.

9 SEIZURE DISORDERS

I. Background

A. Classification

1. **Generalized**
   a. **Grand mal:** Loss of consciousness with symmetric tonic or clonic movements
   b. **Petit mal:** Brief lapses of consciousness
2. **Partial.** Symptoms of seizures reflect area of brain involvement
3. **Unilateral**
4. **Unclassified**
5. When a seizure disorder occurs during pregnancy, the first cause to consider is **eclampsia.** Treat the patient for eclampsia until this diagnosis is ruled out.

B. Incidence. Seizure disorders, the most common neurologic problems of pregnancy, occur at a rate of 1/1,000 pregnancies.

1. 75% of seizures are idiopathic in cause and 25% are organic.
2. 50% of women with seizure disorders will report no change in seizure status during pregnancy.

C. Perinatal Morbidity and Mortality. An increased rate of stillbirths among epileptics on medication has been documented, although the gestational age at which this occurs has not yet been defined.

D. Maternal Morbidity and Mortality. These are the same as in uncomplicated pregnancies.

II. Evaluation

A. History. Did attacks begin in childhood? If she has had a recent seizure, did anyone witness the attack? **Is she currently taking anticonvulsant medications?** Did tongue biting, urinary/fecal incontinence, or a postictal period occur? Is there any history of drug abuse, drug withdrawal, or trauma?

B. Physical Examination. In the patient with recent seizures, pay particular attention to BP, skin (for evidence of trauma), tongue (for evidence of tongue biting during seizure), and the neurologic examination, i.e., deep tendon reflexes.

C. Diagnostic Data

1. If the patient has had a recent seizure,
   a. Obtain serum glucose, calcium (Ca^{++}), magnesium (Mg^{++}), electrolyte panel, and arterial blood gas levels.
   b. Obtain a medication level if she has been taking anticonvulsants.
2. Exclude the diagnosis of eclampsia before initiating anticonvulsant treatment.

III. Therapeutic Management

A. Anticonvulsant Medication

1. A change in the patient's anticonvulsant medications may be made only after consultation with a neurologist.
2. **Phenobarbital** is the drug of choice for a noneclamptic seizure disorder in pregnancy. The average dose of phenobarbital is 100 mg twice daily or three times daily, and the therapeutic level is 10–20 μg/mL. Measure her blood phenobarbital level after she has been taking the medication for 2 weeks.
3. **Phenytoin sodium** (Dilantin) is also used frequently during pregnancy. The average dose is 400 mg/day in a single or divided dose. Up to 1,200 mg/day may be required to maintain a therapeutic blood plasma level of 10–20 μg/mL. (See Chapter 13, section III A1b3 for further details on evaluating dilantin levels.)
4. Monitor **plasma drug levels** carefully.
   a. Anticonvulsant levels require monthly monitoring and adjustment of drug dosages as indicated.
   b. Subtherapeutic plasma drug levels in patients on phenytoin may result from decreased drug absorption and an alternate metabolic pathway.
   c. If seizures continue despite therapeutic medication levels when only one drug (i.e., phenobarbital) is being prescribed, a second drug may be needed.
   d. Anticonvulsant drugs taken during the first trimester

double the infant's risk of a **major congenital malformation** (cleft lip, cleft palate, and congenital heart disease); however, seizures pose a more serious risk to mother and fetus than do anticonvulsant drugs. All medications appear to increase the risk of mental retardation. Some have specific teratogenic effects:

1) **Dilantin** may cause fetal hydantoin syndrome, which consists of craniofacial and limb abnormalities.
2) **Carbamazepine** (Tegretol) may cause craniofacial defects and fingernail hypoplasia.
3) **Valproic acid** (Depakene) may result in fetal neural tube defects.

B. Antepartum Surveillance

1. **Ultrasound evaluation**
   a. Perform an initial scan and fetal echocardiography at 18–20 weeks' gestation to rule out anomalies.
   b. Assess fetal growth through serial scans starting at 26–28 weeks.
2. Start **antepartum testing** at 34 weeks' gestation unless other factors demonstrate an indication for earlier testing.
3. Advise maternal ingestion of **folate,** 1 mg daily.
4. Consider initiating **vitamin K** supplementation (10 mg IM weekly) starting at 34 weeks to prevent neonatal coagulopathy. See also section IIIF.

C. Management of generalized (tonic-clonic) status epilepticus in pregnancy

1. Insert an **IV** line.
2. Draw blood for ethyl alcohol (ETOH) and anticonvulsant drug levels, glucose, BUN, electrolytes, serum Ca^{++}, Mg^{++}, and CBC with differential.
3. Draw an arterial blood sample for **arterial blood gases**; then start O_2 at a high flow rate (8 L/min) by nasal cannula or face mask.
4. Send a urine sample for a **drug screen** (see Appendix R).
5. Perform an **EKG.**
6. Start an IV infusion of normal saline (NS) with B complex. Administer a bolus of 50 ml of 50% glucose, 100 mg thiamine IM.
7. Infuse **diazepam** IV no faster than 5 mg/min until seizures stop (to 40 mg total dose). The duration of diazepam efficacy is only 15–20 minutes, and therefore it is

TABLE 9–1.

Example of Emergency Treatment With **Diazepam** for a Pregnant Patient in Status Epilepticus Weighing 60 kg

1. Push diazepam **10 mg IV** for **2 minutes.**
2. If seizures persist, push an additional 10 mg over 2 minutes.
3. If the patient still does not respond, an additional 20 mg may be used. This provides a **total dose of 40 mg.**
4. **If delivery is imminent;** alert the **pediatrician** (who will be present at the delivery) of the recent diazepam administration—the **infant** will probably be born **depressed** (diazepam has a long half life).

used to abort prolonged episodes and to prevent recurrent convulsions while therapeutic brain concentrations of long-acting anticonvulsants are being achieved.

8. Initiate IV **Dilantin**
   a. Infuse no faster than 50 mg/min, to a total of 18 mg/kg of body weight.
   b. If hypotension develops, slow the infusion rate.
   c. Phenytoin, 50 mg/mL in propylene glycol, may be placed in a 100 ml volume-control set and diluted with NS. Watch the rate of infusion carefully.
   d. Alternatively, phenytoin may be injected slowly by intravenous push (IVP).
   e. Watch for EKG changes:
      1) Atrial and ventricular conduction depression
      2) Ventricular fibrillation
9. **If seizures persist,** an **IV phenobarbital drip** may be initiated.
      1) Insert an endotracheal tube at this time.
      2) Continue to monitor vital signs.
      3) Administer **phenobarbital,** 20 mg/kg maximum, no faster than 100 mg/min, until seizures stop or until a loading dose of **20 mg/kg** is given (Dalessio).

TABLE 9–2.

Example of Emergency Treatment With **Dilantin** for a Pregnant Patient Weighing 60 kg

1. Push **1 g IV** over **20 minutes.**
2. Observe for transient hypotension and heart block.

10. **If seizures continue,** institute general anesthesia with **halothane** and a neuromuscular junction blocker. If an anesthesiologist is not immediately available, give 50–100 mg of **lidocaine** by IVP, slowly.
    1) If lidocaine is effective, administer an IV drip of 50–100 mg diluted in 250 mL of 5% dextrose in water at 1–2 mg/min.
    2) If lidocaine has not stopped the seizures within 20 minutes from the start of the infusion, administer general anesthesia with halothane and a neuromuscular-junction blocker. Continue to monitor vital signs.

D. Management in Labor

1. Patients taking phenobarbital or Dilantin should receive these drugs parenterally. The usual dosages for patients with therapeutic levels are:
   a. **Phenobarbital,** 60 mg IM or IVP (slow) every 6–8 hours.
   b. **Dilantin,** 100 mg IVP every 6–8 hours. Mix only with NS (will precipitate in dextrose).
2. Monitor drug levels if labor is prolonged.
3. Consider administering vitamin K, 10 mg IM.

E. Management Postpartum. Monitor drug levels frequently when the patient is postpartum because of the rapid physiologic changes occurring at this time.

F. Management of the Neonate

1. **Background**
   a. Neonates born to mothers on anticonvulsant therapy (especially barbiturates and phenytoin) are at increased risk of developing clinical or subclinical coagulopathy, even in the absence of coagulopathy in their mothers.
   b. Factors II, VII, IX, and X values are decreased and factors V and VIII values are normal in affected infants (similar to the abnormality produced by a vitamin K deficiency).
2. **Recommendations**
   a. Consider prophylactic administration of vitamin K to the infant after birth.
   b. Measure the prothrombin time (PT) of the cord blood at the time of delivery. If the PT is abnormally low (or clinical evidence of a coagulopathy is present),

treat the infant with fresh frozen plasma (FFP) and IM vitamin K.

BIBLIOGRAPHY

Dalessio DJ: Seizure disorders and pregnancy. *N Engl J Med* 1985; 312:559.

Gabbe SG, Niebyl JR, Simpson JL: *Obstetrics: Normal and Problem Pregnancies*. New York, Churchill Livingstone, 1986.

Jones KL, Lacro RV, Johnson KA, et al: Pattern of malformations in the children of women treated with carbamazepine during pregnancy. *N Engl J Med* 1989; 320:1661.

Kochenour NK, Maurice GE, Sawchuk RJ: Phenytoin metabolism in pregnancy. *Obstet Gynecol* 1980; 56:577.

Nakane Y, Okuma T, Takahashi R, et al: Multi-institutional study in the teratogenicity and fetal toxicity of antiepileptic drugs: A report of a collaborative study group in Japan. *Epilepsia* 1980; 21:663.

Nelson KB, Ellenberg JH: Maternal seizure disorder, outcome of pregnancy and neurologic abnormalities in the children. *Neurology* 1982; 32:1247.

Orland MJ, Saltmeir RJ: *Manual of Medical Therapeutics,* Boston, Little Brown, 1986.

URINARY TRACT INFECTIONS 10

I. Background

A. Definitions

1. **Asymptomatic bacteriuria (ASB)** is the presence of $>10^5$ bacteria/mL of urine in a patient who is asymptomatic for a urinary tract infection.
   a. **Incidence.** 2% to 8% of women have an ASB. This is not increased during pregnancy.
   b. 20% to 40% of pregnant patients with ASB will develop acute pyelonephritis if the ASB is not treated.
2. **Cystitis** is significant bacteriuria accompanied by urinary urgency, polyuria, and dysuria, without fever or costovertebral angle tenderness.
3. **Pyelonephritis** is the presence of significant bacteriuria in the upper urinary tract, often with symptoms of chills, fever, and sometimes lower urinary tract infection.
   a. **Incidence**
      1) Pyelonephritis occurs in 1%–2% of pregnant women.
      2) Pyelonephritis may be prevented in 60%–70% of patients by screening for ASB and rendering appropriate treatment.
      3) Pyelonephritis develops more frequently from an ASB during pregnancy because of urinary stasis in the renal pelvis (which dilates in response to the elevated progesterone during pregnancy or from pressure on the ureters from the gravid uterus).
   b. The **pathogen** is *Escherichia* coli in 85% of patients, while the remaining infections are caused by *Klebsiella, Proteus,* enterococcus, staphylococcus, and group D streptococci.

c. Pyelonephritis is right sided in 85% of patients and left sided in 15%.

II. Evaluation of Patients With Pyelonephritis

A. **History.** The patient may complain of dysuria, frequency, back pain, chills, fever, nausea, vomiting, or uterine contractions. Rule out preterm labor in these patients.

B. **Physical Examination.** Perform a thorough physical examination. Pay particular attention to the patient's temperature curve and other vital signs, costovertebral angle tenderness, and abdominal examination. (Are uterine contractions appreciated? Is her uterus tender?)

C. **Diagnostic Data**

1. Obtain:
   a. **Urinalysis** with **culture and sensitivity** (C&S) and Gram's stain of unspun urine. If these studies were previously sent from the office, the results may be ready for evaluation at the time the patient presents to Labor and Delivery for evaluation.
   b. **CBC with differential**
2. Review the patient's prenatal laboratory tests for a previous ASB with a documented C&S to guide current therapy.

D. The **differential diagnosis** includes appendicitis, ruptured ovarian cyst, and cholecystitis. Refer to Chapter 3 for an evaluation of abdominal pain in pregnancy.

III. Therapeutic Management of Patients With Pyelonephritis

A. Obtain a catheterized urine sample before treatment is initiated. Do not allow the urine to sit at room temperature. Send the specimen on ice if transport is delayed. Note on the laboratory slip the date and time that the specimen was obtained.

B. Antibiotic therapy will vary according to the specific sensitivity of the causative organisms at your facility and according to the patient's clinical status. Suggestions for initiating treatment are detailed here.

1. The patient who appears hemodynamically stable may be started on cephapirin sodium **(Cefadyl),** 2 g, intravenous piggyback every 6 hours, or **ampicillin,** 2 g, intravenous piggyback every 4 hours.
2. For the patient who appears toxic (high fever, chills,

tachycardia), initiate therapy with **ampicillin** (for gram-positive coverage) and **gentamicin** (for gram-negative coverage).

3. After a few days when her condition has stabilized, she is afebrile, and her urine C&S results are obtained, consider discontinuing one of the antibiotics.

C. If results of the C&S warrant, or if the patient has not responded to therapy within 48 hours, consider changing antibiotics.

D. Continue IV antibiotics for up to **5 days** or until she is **afebrile for 48 hours,** whichever occurs first. An oral antibiotic may then be initiated to complete a 10-day course. Commonly used oral antibiotics include:

1. Cefaclor (Ceclor), 500 mg every 6 hours
2. Nitrofurantoin, 100 mg every 6 hours
3. Ampicillin, 500 mg every 6 hours
4. Others per sensitivity studies

E. If at 96 hours the patient is still febrile, **a ureteral obstruction** may be present. Obtain a renal ultrasound evaluation to look for renal stones and anomalies. If a distal ureteral stone cannot be ruled out, obtain a single-shot intravenous pyelogram.

F. To assure **adequate hydration,** encourage a large fluid intake (3–4 L/day minimum).

G. Place the patient in **semi-Fowler's position** on the side opposite the affected kidney.

H. Obtain a **catheterized urine specimen** for analysis, Gram's stain, and C&S **48 hours after admission.** Before discharge, the patient must have at least a negative Gram's stain, with culture pending, although negative culture results are preferable.

I. Reevaluate the patient in the office within 1 week.

J. If the patient has a **second course of pyelonephritis** during this pregnancy, place her on **antibiotic suppression** (daily oral nitrofurantoin, 100 mg) after completing a full antibiotic treatment course. Continue the antibiotic suppression until 6 weeks' postpartum.

K. Consider obtaining an intravenous pyelogram **6 weeks postpartum** if the patient had either left-sided pyelonephritis, or more than one episode of pyelonephritis, during her pregnancy.

L. Urine cultures should be obtained monthly on all patients with an episode of antepartum pyelonephritis.

BIBLIOGRAPHY

American College of Obstetricians and Gynecologists: *Antimicrobial Therapy for Obstetric Patients*. Technical Bulletin No. 117, ACOG, Washington DC, 1988.

Duff P: Pyelonephritis in pregnancy. *Clin Obstet Gynecol* 1984; 27:17.

Part III

OBSTETRIC COMPLICATIONS

HYPEREMESIS GRAVIDARUM — 11

I. Background

A. Definition. Hyperemesis gravidarum is persistent vomiting unresponsive to outpatient therapy and severe enough to cause acetonuria, dehydration, electrolyte imbalances, weight loss (or all of these) in the first trimester.

B. Incidence. Hyperemesis gravidarum occurs in 3.5 of 1,000 pregnancies.

C. Etiology

1. Elevated estradiol and human chorionic gonadotropin levels are most likely related to the cause of hyperemesis gravidarum. Various studies have demonstrated higher estradiol levels in women who are nulliparous, in the first trimester of their first pregnancy, or are heavyset. Cigarette smoking has been shown to decrease estrogen levels. Human chorionic gonadotropin level is known to be elevated in patients with multiple gestations.
2. The profile of patients with hyperemesis gravidarum includes those who are younger, nulliparous, heavyset, and have multiple gestations. In addition, patients with hyperemesis gravidarum are less likely to smoke cigarettes and are more likely to have more years of education than those who do not have any form of emesis resulting from pregnancy.

D. Differential Diagnosis. Pancreatitis, hepatitis, cholelithiasis, cholecystitis, peptic ulcer, pneumonia, hyperthyroidism, intestinal or ovarian torsion, volvulus, appendicitis, diabetes mellitus, and a brain tumor

E. Perinatal Morbidity and Mortality

1. Both hyperemesis gravidarum and the less severe nausea and vomiting during pregnancy have been associated

with a good pregnancy outcome and a low spontaneous abortion rate.
2. Antiemetics do not appear to be teratogenic.
3. Patients with true hyperemesis gravidarum with weight loss and electrolyte disturbances have demonstrated a statistically significant increase in intrauterine growth retardation. (Thus these fetuses should be monitored carefully for appropriate weight gain.)

F. Maternal Morbidity and Mortality. The primary morbidity caused by this disorder is the need for recurrent hospitalizations. Otherwise maternal morbidity and mortality are unchanged from those of uncomplicated pregnancies.

II. Evaluation

A. History. Quantify the amount of vomiting and its temporal relation to meals, physical activity, illness, stress, and emotional trauma (desire for pregnancy, response to pregnancy, support of husband or mate).

B. Physical Examination. A thorough physical examination must be performed to rule out other causes of nausea in pregnancy.

1. Inspect the skin for turgor, the tongue for furrowing, the thyroid gland for enlargement and nodularity, the lungs for evidence of infection, and the abdomen for evidence of peritoneal irritation.
2. If pain or tenderness is present, evaluate its location, radiation, and severity. Gastrointestinal disorders present differently during pregnancy. (Please refer to Chapter 3 for further details on evaluating abdominal pain in pregnancy.)
3. Observe the vomitus for color, amount, consistency. (Is it true vomitus or saliva?)

C. Diagnostic Data. Obtain a blood glucose and electrolyte panel, amylase or diastase, prothrombin time, CBC with differential, urinalysis to look for ketones (if present, obtain a serum acetone test) and specific gravity (to evaluate overall fluid status), and a stool Hemoccult.

III. Therapeutic Management

A. Outpatient

1. For patients with **mild** symptoms without significant starvation and dehydration, follow instructions in Table 11–1.

TABLE 11–1.
Dietary Instructions for Patient With Hyperemesis Gravidarum

Keep a supply of crackers at the bedside, and eat a few of these upon awakening in the morning, before getting out of bed.
Eat approximately six small high-protein meals a day.
Ice chips and liquids (including weak teas and colas) may be taken between meals, but minimize fluid intake with meals.
Avoid substances irritating to the intestinal tract.
Adhere to the preceding recommendations as closely as possible for resolution of nausea.

2. Patients with **moderate** symptoms, or those who were previously instructed to follow the recommendations in Table 11–1 but now return with persistent symptoms, may be treated pharmacologically.
   a. **Intravenous hydration** may be provided if indicated.
   b. **Antihistamines,** such as **promethazine** (Phenergan) 25 mg orally (po) every 4 to 6 hours, and **doxylamine succinate** (Decapryn, Unisom), 25 mg po at bedtime (hs) and in the morning as needed (prn), may be prescribed with or without **vitamin B_6,** 10–50 mg po daily. Inform the patient that drowsiness may be a side effect of antihistamines.
3. Patients with **persistent symptoms** despite treatment, as has been detailed, may be hydrated intravenously and treated with the following:
   a. **Phenothiazines** (dopamine antagonists) such as
      1) **Prochlorperazine** (Compazine), 10 mg IM or po, or 25 mg suppository per rectum every 8 hours prn, **or**
      2) **Metoclopramide** (Reglan), 10 mg po after every other meal (for patients adhering to six small meals a day) and at hs, or prn.
      3) Side effects of both of these medications include extrapyramidal symptoms (EPS), primarily dystonic and akathisia reactions.
   b. **Diphenhydramine** (Benadryl), 25–50 mg po every 8 hours may be used in conjunction with the phenothiazines, and may prevent EPS.

B. Inpatient. Hospitalization is indicated when outpatient management fails.
   1. Hydrate and correct electrolyte imbalances.

2. Provide antiemetics (for the obvious as well as sedation).
3. **Compazine,** 10 mg IM or 25 mg suppositories every 6 hours. Concurrent use of **Benadryl,** 50 mg every 8 hours po, IM, or IV, may prevent EPS from Compazine. Decrease to 25 mg every 6 hours as indicated by the patient's sedation level.
4. **Hydroxyzine pamoate** (Vistaril), 50 mg IM or po every 4 hours.
5. **Droperidol** (Inapsine), a butyrophenone (dopamine antagonist), is more potent than the phenothiazines, and has fewer cardiovascular, respiratory, and EPS side effects. It may be administered as:
   a. 2.5 mg IM or IV every 6 hours **or**
   b. A **continuous infusion** of 25 mg in 500 mL 5% dextrose in water (0.05 mg/mL). Run in a 2.5 mg bolus; then set at 1 mg (20 mL) per hour.
6. Bed rest with privacy is desirable, with dietary restrictions until the patient recovers (usually 24 hours).
7. When nausea resolves, initiate a diet with small frequent meals, as detailed in Table 11–1. Consultation with a dietitian is recommended.
8. If the patient is unable to tolerate any amount of oral intake for several days, **hyperalimentation** may avoid the need for prolonged recurrent hospitalization.
9. **Upon recovery,** intravenous antiemetics may be discontinued and oral therapy initiated. **Oral Reglan** (10 mg) and **Vistaril** (50 mg) are to be used concurrently, with administration of each a half hour before every other meal (if the patient is eating six small meals a day) and at bedtime (for a total of four doses of each medication daily). Discontinue Inapsine at least 60 minutes before initiating oral antiemetic therapy.
10. A **team approach** to the patient's care is recommended, with involvement of nursing personnel experienced in the care of patients with hyperemesis as well as involvement of dietary and social service personnel. Upon discharge from the hospital, initiate telephone contact with the patient (at least once before her next office visit) for positive reassurance and encouragement of adherence to the dietary guidelines.
11. The patient is to return to the office within 1 week from discharge.

Acknowledgment

Droperidol administration instructions courtesy of Gerald G. Briggs, B.Pharm., Long Beach Memorial Medical Center, Long Beach, Calif.

BIBLIOGRAPHY

Gross S, Librach C, Cecutti A: Maternal weight loss associated with hyperemesis gravidarum: A predictor of fetal outcome. *Am J Obstet Gynecol* 1989; 160:906–909.

Niebyl JR: Therapeutic drugs in pregnancy: Caution is the watchword. *Postgrad Med* 1984; 75:165–172.

INCOMPETENT CERVIX 12

I. Backround

A. **Definition.** Incompetent cervix is a condition in which the cervix is physically inadequate, spontaneously dilating at or beyond 16 weeks' gestation, with a resultant premature pregnancy loss.

B. **Incidence.** Cervical incompetence occurs in 0.05%–1% of all pregnancies and is responsible for 15%–20% of second-trimester pregnancy losses.

C. **Etiology**

1. **Cervical trauma**
   a. Dilation (diagnostic curettage or elective abortion)
   b. Conization
   c. Laceration after a precipitous or operative vaginal delivery
   d. Cervical amputation (archaic treatment for uterine prolapse)
2. **Congenital**
   a. Associated with uterine anomalies
   b. In utero diethylstilbestrol exposure
   c. Increased cervical muscular composition with resultant decreased inherent cervical resistance

D. **Pathophysiology.** The region of incompetence is postulated to be the site of cervical resistance, not the cervical isthmus, which is completely distended by 20 weeks' gestation. As the collagen concentration of the cervix declines in proportion to an increase in the muscular content, cervical resistance is lowered, and an increase in incompetence is noted.

II. Antenatal Evaluation (of a patient with a prior second-trimester pregnancy loss)

A. The patient's **obstetric history** is extremely important in diagnosing this disorder.

1. Inquire as to whether a **classic** or **nonclassic presentation** for cervical incompetence was present before the spontaneous abortion.
2. The **classic presentation** of a patient with cervical incompetence is a history of one or more spontaneous abortions between 14 and 28 weeks' gestation. Generally the patient has an uneventful pregnancy until the mid second trimester. At this time painless cervical effacement and dilation occur, with a watery discharge and bulging of the membranes (creating a vague abdominal/pelvic pressure). Typically, contractions are absent until late in the process. Eventually the membranes rupture, followed by abortion.
3. A **nonclassical presentation** is much more difficult to diagnose accurately. Here, the patient may present with atypical preterm labor. Uterine contractions may be present, but occur once every 10 to 15 minutes. The cervix is dilated despite very mild uterine activity. In addition, the cervix may appear to fall open despite a very gentle examination. A suspicion of cervical incompetence must be high when a patient presents in this manner.
4. Ask the patient about the etiologic factors detailed in section IC1.

B. Perform a **physical examination.** Inspect the cervix for anomalies and prior trauma.

C. Diagnostic Data

1. No objective criteria are available to establish the diagnosis of cervical incompetence in the nonpregnant state. Previously, attempts were made at using hysterosalpingograms and cervical dilators to detect incompetence, but the data were unreliable.
2. More recently, early pregnancy ultrasound has been applied to assist in this diagnosis. The diagnostic value of ultrasound in nonclassical cervical incompetence has been limited.

III. Second-Trimester Evaluation Upon Presentation to Emergency Room

A. History. Inquire into the patient's symptoms.

1. Was her pregnancy uneventful until this time? Has she

had any known recent cervical infections? Has she felt contractions? Ruptured her membranes?

2. Does she have any risk factors (cervical trauma, congenital etiology [listed previously], or a previous episode of a second-trimester loss thought to result from cervical incompetence)?

B. Physical Examination. Perform a thorough physical examination. Evaluate the cervix for dilation and effacement. It is difficult to inspect the cervix for anomalies and prior trauma at this time.

C. Diagnostic Data

1. Monitor the uterus for contractions.
2. If contractions are present, rule out preterm labor.

IV. Therapeutic Management. Surgery is the primary treatment for an incompetent cervix (Table 12–1).

A. In a nonpregnant woman with a strong history of an incompetent cervix, search for an anatomic defect during the **physical examination.** If a substantial defect is present, consider a primary repair (i.e., Lash procedure, or cerclage at the uterosacral-cardinal ligaments, as indicated). If no anatomic abnormality is present, prophylactically place a cerclage at 14–16 weeks' gestation in her next pregnancy.

B. In a patient presenting for a **routine prenatal examination in the first trimester** with a history suggestive of an incompetent cervix, consider placing a cerclage prophylactically at 14–16 weeks' gestation. Weekly cervical examinations may be done to assess cervical dilation in the first few weeks of the second trimester, before the planned procedure. The McDonald and Shirodkar techniques are the most commonly performed cerclage procedures in this setting.

C. When cervical incompetence is **diagnosed during pregnancy:**

1. Place the patient in the **Trendelenburg position** (at least 10 degrees). If the membranes have prolapsed into the vagina, Trendelenburg positioning may allow them to recede back into the uterine cavity.
2. Patients ineligible for cerclage placement, or those who refuse the procedure, have very poor pregnancy outcomes. An abortion often occurs imminently.
3. Placement of a **cervical cerclage** is available to patients

TABLE 12–1.

Treatment Modalities for the Incompetent Cervix

Procedure	Indication	Timing	Notes	Complications
Lash	Anatomic defect caused by cervical trauma	Nonpregnant state	Repair of anatomic defect	Infertility (rarely)
Shirodkar	Cervical incompetence	Nonpregnant or 14–16 weeks' gestation	Placement of a 5 mm Mersilene band at level of internal os; bladder is advanced off the cervix	Hemorrhage, cervical dystocia, PROM, chorioamnionitis, placental abscess, uterine rupture, maternal death
McDonald	Useful when lower uterine segment is significantly effaced	Nonpregnant or 14–16 weeks' gestation	Placement of a 5 mm Mersilene band or other permanent suture in a purse-string fashion high on the cervix	Hemorrhage, cervical dystocia, PROM, chorioamnionitis, placental abscess, uterine rupture, maternal death

Uterosacral cardinal ligament cerclage	Amputated or congenitally short cervix; subacute cervicitis; previous failed Shirodkar or McDonald cerclage	Nonpregnant	Intra-abdominal and vaginal procedures are possible; cesarean delivery is mandatory	Hemorrhage, cervical dystocia, PROM, chorioamnionitis, placental abscess, uterine rupture, maternal death
Hefner	Well-developed lower uterine segment with minimal cervix remaining	Late diagnosis of incompetence	Mattress or U sutures	Hemorrhage, cervical dystocia, PROM, chorioamnionitis, placental abscess, uterine rupture, maternal death

PROM = premature rupture of membranes.

without the contraindications listed below. A McDonald cerclage is the most commonly used surgical procedure for treatment of cervical incompetence during pregnancy. Before cerclage placement, obtain cervical cultures for gonorrhea and group B β-streptococcus. The optimal time to place a cerclage is between 14 and 16 weeks' gestation. If the gestation is more than 20 weeks, the success rate dramatically decreases.

a. **Contraindications to Cervical Cerclage**
   1) Hyperirritability of the uterus, with bulging membranes
   2) Cervical dilatation >4 cm
   3) Fetal malformation or demise
   4) Premature rupture of membranes (PROM)

b. **Complications of Cervical Cerclage**
   1) PROM (1%–9%)
   2) Chorioamnionitis (1%–7%)
      The risk of PROM and chorioamnionitis for an elective cerclage at the beginning of the second trimester is less than 1%. The risk increases as the pregnancy progresses. When the cervix is dilated more than 3 cm, with prolapsed membranes, a 30% risk of rupture of the membranes or chorioamnionitis (or both) is present.
   3) Preterm labor
   4) Cervical laceration or amputation (This may occur during the procedure, or at delivery. A band of scar tissue may form on the cervix at the site of the suture, resulting in failure to progress or a cervical laceration.)
   5) Bladder injury (rare)

c. In addition to the standard **surgical technique** of cerclage placement, consider:
   1) **Spinal conduction anesthesia** (to prevent maternal straining)
   2) **Filling the bladder** via a Foley catheter with approximately 500–1,000 mL of normal saline or sterile water (This will assist in elevating the membranes off the cervix.)
   3) **Antibiotic prophylaxis** of chorioamnionitis (especially for gestations beyond 18 weeks) for 2–3 days after the cerclage placement (i.e., ampicillin,

2 g, intravenous piggyback every 6 hours for 3 days)

4) Administration of **indomethacin** (Indocin), 50 mg (orally or rectally) before the procedure and 25 mg every 6 hours for one or two additional doses after the procedure (to block the prostaglandins that will be released during the procedure)

d. **Postoperative Care**

1) It is important that the patient is at bed rest for 24 hours and is observed for increased uterine activity.
2) The patient is to have pelvic rest for the remainder of her pregnancy, together with limited physical activity with frequent rest periods each day.
3) If increased uterine activity occurs, consider tocolysis, depending on the gestational age of the fetus.
4) The patient is to be seen weekly in the office.
5) Instruct the patient in the early signs and symptoms of chorioamnionitis. Have her monitor her temperature daily and return immediately to the office or hospital if any signs of infection develop.
6) Consider removal of the cerclage if she subsequently prematurely ruptures her chorioamniotic membranes.
7) Remove the cerclage electively at 37 weeks' gestation in the office if her antepartum course has not required earlier removal.
8) Provide preterm labor education, including precautions.

e. **Success:** It is difficult to define the true success of a cerclage because data concerning the recurrence rate of cervical incompetence are lacking. It is stated that 80%–90% of pregnancies in which a cerclage is placed have resulted in live, viable births. Eighty-five percent of patients with one previous preterm birth and 70% with two preterm births will deliver at term.

BIBLIOGRAPHY

Chryssikopoulos DB, Botsis D, Vitoratos N, et al: Cervical incompetence: A 24 year review. *Int J Gynecol Obstet* 1988; 26:245–253.

Cousins L: Cervical incompetence 1980: A time for reappraisal. *Clin Obstet Gynecol* 1980; 23:467.

Gabbe SG, Niebyl JR, Simpson JL: *Obstetrics: Normal and Problem Pregnancies*. New York, Churchill Livingstone, 1986.

Goodlin RC: Surgical treatment of patients with hour glass shaped or ruptured membranes prior to the twenty-fifth week of gestation. *Surg Gynecol Obstet* 1987; 165:410–412.

Scheerer LJ, Lam F, Bartolucci L, et al: A new technique for reduction of prolapsed fetal membranes for emergency cervical cerclage. *Obstet Gynecol* 1989; 74:408–410.

Yeast JD, Garite TJ: The role of cervical cerclage in the management of preterm premature rupture of membranes. *Am J Obstet Gynecol* 1988; 158:106–110.

CHORIOAMNIONITIS 13

I. Background

A. Definition

1. Chorioamnionitis is a clinical syndrome of intra-amniotic infection associated with acute inflammation of the fetal membranes, which is clinically manifested before delivery.
2. By convention, if the clinical syndrome resolves within the first 24 hours after delivery, chorioamnionitis is the only diagnosis; however, if the fever, uterine tenderness, and other signs of infection persist beyond this time, the patient now has the additional complication of **endometritis** or **endomyometritis.**

B. Incidence. Chorioamnionitis occurs in 0.5%–1.0% of all pregnancies and in 3%–25% of patients with premature rupture of membranes (PROM) lasting longer than 24 hours.

C. Etiology. Infection ascends either through intact or (more commonly) ruptured membranes, transplacentally, or descends from the abdominal cavity through the fallopian tubes (rare).

D. Perinatal Morbidity and Mortality. In the presence of chorioamnionitis, sepsis will occur in the fetus or neonate at term in about 5% of cases. In the preterm gestation, approximately 20%–25% of neonates will have serious infectious complications.

E. Maternal Morbidity and Mortality. Maternal complications include preterm labor and endometritis. If sepsis occurs, any of its sequelae may result, such as acute respiratory distress syndrome, renal failure, disseminated intravascular coagulation, and shock.

F. Risk Factors. Amniocentesis, PROM, repetitive vaginal examinations, internal fetal heart rate monitoring.

II. Evaluation

A. History. Elicit information pertaining to membrane rupture, recent amniocentesis, and repetitive vaginal examinations because the most common route of infection, after PROM, is transvaginally.

B. Physical Examination

1. Maternal fever is seen in almost all patients with chorioamnionitis.
2. About one fifth demonstrate foul-smelling amniotic fluid.
3. Uterine tenderness is noted in a minority of patients.
4. A thorough fever workup should be conducted for all patients with suspected chorioamnionitis so that the potential causes of febrile morbidity are not missed. Rule out other sources of infection, such as the upper respiratory tract, urinary tract, and abdomen (see Chapter 3).

C. Diagnostic Data

1. In the presence of ruptured membranes, the diagnosis of chorioamnionitis is made in the presence of fever (≥38° C) and one or more of the following:
   a. Uterine tenderness
   b. WBC >18,000
   c. Fetal tachycardia
   d. Foul-smelling vaginal effluent
2. In patients with intact membranes and an unexplained fever (especially in the presence of preterm labor), amniocentesis may be necessary to confirm the diagnosis. In the presence of clinically apparent chorioamnionitis, amniocentesis should reveal both leukocytes and bacteria to be consistent with the diagnosis.
3. In patients at term in labor, fluid may be withdrawn from an intrauterine pressure catheter and sent to the lab for Gram's staining (this will aid in early confirmation of the diagnosis and identifying the causative organism) and culture.
4. Vaginal and cervical cultures are of little help in the evaluation of chorioamnionitis.

III. Therapeutic Management

A. The basic management of chorioamnionitis includes delivery and the administration of antibiotics. There is no place for expectant management; after the diagnosis is made, delivery must follow regardless of gestational age.

B. The diagnosis of chorioamnionitis should not affect the route of delivery. If the patient is otherwise a candidate for vaginal delivery and is not in labor, labor is induced. If she is in labor, cesarean section is reserved for the usual obstetric indications, and the duration of labor allowed is not altered.

C. Generally, after the diagnosis of chorioamnionitis is made, antibiotics should be started. One possible exception is the patient who has a clinically mild infection and whose delivery is expected imminently (<1 hour).

D. Antibiotic choices may vary from institution to institution, but reasonable choices include **ampicillin,** a **cephalosporin,** or a semisynthetic antibiotic such as ampicillin with a β-lactamase inhibitor (i.e., sulbactam [Unasyn]). In the patient who is clinically toxic (i.e., high fever, marked tachycardia, rigors), an **aminoglycoside** should be added.

E. In the presence of chorioamnionitis and maternal fever, the fetus is expected to be tachycardic. This is not indicative of fetal distress in and of itself, and is not an indication for cesarean section.

F. After delivery, antibiotics are generally continued for at least 24 hours. Many patients will defervesce immediately postpartum, and antibiotics can be discontinued completely in these patients at 24 hours. If the fever is persistent after delivery, the patient should have antibiotics continued as in patients with endometritis.

BIBLIOGRAPHY

Garite TJ, Freeman RK: Chorioamnionitis in the preterm gestation. *Am J Obstet Gynecol* 1982; 59:539–545.

Gibbs RS, Castillo MS, Rodgers PJ: Management of acute chorioamnionitis. *Am J Obstet Gynecol* 1980; 136:709–713.

Gibbs RS, Dinsmoor MJ, Newton ER, et al: A randomized trial of intrapartum versus immediate postpartum treatment of women with intra-amniotic infection. *Obstet Gynecol* 1988; 72:825–828.

Romero R, Sirtori M, Oyarzun E, et al: Infection and labor. V: Prevalence, microbiology, and clinical significance of intraamniotic infection in women with preterm labor and intact membranes. *Am J Obstet Gynecol* 1989; 161:817–824.

Skoll MA, Moretti ML, Sibai BM: The incidence of positive amniotic fluid cultures in patients with preterm labor with intact membranes. *Am J Obstet Gynecol* 1989; 161:813–816.

PREMATURE RUPTURE OF THE FETAL MEMBRANES

14

I. Background

A. **Definition.** Premature rupture of membranes (PROM) is the spontaneous rupture of the chorioamniotic membrane at any time before the onset of labor. The definition does not imply gestational age.
   1. **Preterm PROM** is rupture before 36 weeks.
   2. **Prolonged** rupture of the membranes is rupture for more than 24 hours.

B. **Incidence.** PROM occurs in 8.1%–18.5% of pregnancies, with an average of about 12%.

C. **Etiology.** The cause of PROM is usually unknown. At term, PROM may be a physiologic event. Preterm PROM is often thought to be due to an occult chorioamnionitis. Infrequent identifiable causes include:
   1. Polyhydramnios
   2. Incompetent cervix
   3. Amniocentesis
   4. Trauma (rarely)

II. Perinatal and Maternal Morbidity

A. **Labor** usually follows PROM within a relatively short time (90% within 24 hours at term). If preterm PROM occurs, **premature labor and delivery** is the most common complication.

B. **Infection,** either maternal (chorioamnionitis) or fetal (i.e., sepsis, pneumonia) may occur as a result of ascending vaginal infection after PROM or if an occult intra-amniotic infection preceded the rupture of membranes (ROM).

C. **Umbilical cord compression** may result from oligohydramnios resulting from PROM. This may occur antepartum or intrapartum, and, if severe, may result in asphyxia or fetal death.

D. **Abruptio placentae** occurs more frequently in the presence of PROM.

E. **Fetal deformation syndrome** may occur in the very premature gestation with prolonged ROM and marked oligohydramnios. This includes intrauterine growth retardation, pulmonary hypoplasia, and limb deformities due to compression.

III. Patient Evaluation

A. **History.** A typical history includes a large gush of fluid from the vagina, with subsequent continued leakage. A consistent history correctly identifies the diagnosis more than 90% of the time.

B. **Physical Examination**

1. **Avoid digital examination of the cervix** in patients not in apparent active labor, because this examination markedly increases the risk of infection.
2. **Diagnosis**
   a. In patients with a history suggestive of PROM, the diagnosis is confirmed by **aseptic speculum examination,** at which at least two of the following criteria are noted:
      1) **Pooling.** A pool of fluid is visible in the posterior fornix.
      2) **Phenaphthazine** (Nitrazine). Yellow Nitrazine paper turns **dark blue** in the presence of alkaline amniotic fluid.
      3) **Ferning.** A smear of fluid from the vaginal fornix creates a typical fern pattern if amniotic fluid is present.
      4) **Oligohydramnios.** Ultrasound showing little or no amniotic fluid is consistent with PROM.

   b. Evaluate the patient to **rule out infection.** Pay particular attention to the following:
      1) Fever
      2) Tender uterus

3) Foul-smelling amniotic fluid leaking from the vagina
4) Fetal tachycardia
5) Leukocytosis

c. **Rule out fetal distress:**
1) **Prolonged fetal monitoring** (12–24 hours) in labor and delivery is recommended upon admission to the hospital.
2) Follow with a **daily nonstress test** to rule out cord compression if the patient is placed on expectant management.

d. Evaluate the **gestational age** and **fetal maturity:**
1) Carefully review the patient's dating criteria.
2) Obtain ultrasound biometry.
3) If the period of gestation is ≥33 weeks, consider obtaining fetal lung maturity testing by:
   a) Amniocentesis (lecithin/sphingomyelin ratio or other tests)
   b) Fluid collection from the vagina may be reliably tested for phosphatidyglycerol.

IV. Therapeutic Management

A. Overview
1. The management of PROM is very controversial, and approaches will vary from institution to institution.
2. Three variables enter into the basic management decision of whether to deliver immediately or await the spontaneous onset of labor:
   a. Gestational age
   b. Concern regarding increased risk of infection as the duration of ROM becomes prolonged
   c. Increased likelihood of cesarean section with induction of labor

B. Options for Management of a Term Gestation
1. **Active Management.** Begin oxytocin induction upon admission.
2. **Expectant Management.** Await the spontaneous onset of labor and intervene sooner only for clinical infection, fetal distress, or other obstetric indications.
3. **Other Intermediate Options**
   a. **Delayed Active Management.** Allow a reasonable

time (i.e., 24 hours) for spontaneous labor and then begin oxytocin if labor does not ensue.

b. Administer preinduction prostaglandin followed by **induction** with oxytocin.

C. **Options for Management of a Preterm Gestation**

1. Most use some form of **expectant management** in preterm gestations awaiting spontaneous labor and delivering sooner only for fetal distress, infection, or other obstetric indications.
2. Variations
   a. **Tocolysis.** Some use tocolytics for preterm labor in PROM, but evidence of benefit is lacking.
   b. **Corticosteroids.** While these clearly accelerate lung maturity in premature labor, in the face of PROM there is little evidence of benefit.
   c. **Antibiotics.** Prophylactic antibiotics show great promise for patients with PROM, but these data are new and the practice is not yet common.
   d. **Selective Active Management**
      1) Delivery for patients with amniotic fluid testing indicating fetal maturity
      2) Delivery for patients with amniotic fluid Gram's stain indicating occult infection (fluid obtained by amniocentesis only)

BIBLIOGRAPHY

American College of Obstetricians and Gynecologists: *Management of Premature Rupture of Membranes*. Technical Bulletin No. 115, April 1988.

Garite TJ: Premature rupture of membranes. *Curr Probl Obstet Gynecol* 1984; 7:671–679.

Gibbs RS, Blanco JD: Premature rupture of membranes. *Obstet Gynecol* 1982; 60:671.

Ohlsson A: Treatment of preterm premature rupture of membranes: A meta-analysis. *Am J Obstet Gynecol* 1989; 160:890–906.

Veille JC: Management of preterm premature rupture of membranes. *Am J Obstet Gynecol* 1987; 157:851–863.

PRETERM LABOR 15

I. Background

A. Definition. Preterm labor **(PTL)** is present when at least one regular contraction occurs every 10 minutes in the presence of cervical effacement or dilatation. The rate of error in diagnosis is 50%.

B. Incidence. PTL occurs in 8%–10% of all pregnancies. The recurrence rate is 25%–50%. Those patients at highest risk are identified by the premature labor risk assessment (Table 15–1).

C. The **etiology** is multifactorial:

1. Premature rupture of membranes (PROM), 38%
2. Idiopathic, 30%
3. Abruption/previa, 15%
4. Amnionitis, 7%
5. Miscellaneous, 10%

D. Perinatal Morbidity and Mortality. Premature labor accounts for 50%–75% of all perinatal morbidity and mortality, if delivery occurs.

E. Maternal Morbidity and Mortality. Maternal morbidity and mortality are the same as that noted in uncomplicated pregnancies.

F. The **risk factors** for PTL may be divided into major and minor categories. Refer to Table 15–2 for further details.

II. Evaluation

A. History

1. The patient will often complain of lower back pain, pelvic pressure, vaginal discharge, loose stools, spotting, and menstrual-like cramps. Inquire as to the duration of the symptoms present.
2. Identify precipitating factors such as trauma, emesis, diarrhea, urinary tract infection, and PROM.

TABLE 15–1.

Premature Labor—Risk Evaluation*

Points†	Socioeconomic Status	Past History	Daily Habits	Current Pregnancy
1	2 children at home Low socioeconomic status	1 abortion Less thay 1 yr since last birth	Work outside home	Unusual fatigue
2	Younger than 20 yr Older than 40 yr Single parent	2 abortions	More than 10 cigarettes per day	Less than 4.0 kg gain by 32 wk gestation Albuminuria Hypertension Bacteriuria
3	Very low socioeconomic status Shorter than 150 cm Lighter than 45 kg	3 abortions	Heavy work; long, tiring trip	Breech at 32 wk Weight loss of 2 kg Head engaged Febrile illness

4	Younger than 18 yr	Pyelonephritis		Metrorrhagia after 12 wk gestation Effacement Dilatation Uterine irritability
5		Uterine anomaly Second-trimester abortion DES exposure		Placenta previa Hydramnios
10		Premature delivery Repeated second-trimester abortion		Twins Abdominal surgery

DES = diethylstilbestrol.

*From Creasy RK, Gummer BA, Liggins GC: *Obstet Gynecol* 1980; 55:692. As published in Main DM, Main EK: *Obstetrics and Gynecology. A Pocket Reference.* St Louis, Mosby–Year Book, 1984. Used by permission.

†Score is computed by addition of the number of points given any item. 0–5 = low risk; 6–9 = medium risk; 10 or more = high risk. In this study 9% of patients were high risk for premature delivery on initial screening; one third of these patients delivered prematurely, accounting for two thirds of all the premature infants delivered. Rescoring at 26–28 wk gestation improves the accuracy of the prediction.

TABLE 15–2.
Major and Minor Risk Factors in Prediction of Spontaneous Preterm Labor*

Major Risk Factors†	Minor Risk Factors†
Multiple gestation	Febrile illness
DES exposure	Bleeding after 12 wk
Hydramnios	History of pyelonephritis
Uterine anomaly	Cigarettes—more than 10/day
Cervix dilated >1 cm at 32 wk	Second-trimester abortion ×1
Second-trimester abortion ×2	More than 2 first-trimester abortions
Previous preterm delivery	
Previous preterm labor; term delivery	
Abdominal surgery during pregnancy	
History of cone biopsy	
Cervical shortening <1 cm at 32 wk	
Uterine irritability	

*Adapted from Creasy RK, Resnick R: *Maternal-Fetal Medicine.* Philadelphia, WB Saunders, 1984, p 481.
†The presence of one or more major factors or two or more minor factors (or both) places the patient in a high-risk group for preterm labor.
DES = diethylstilbestrol.

B. Upon admission, a thorough **physical examination** is mandatory. When taking vital signs, pay particular attention to the patient's temperature and BP. During the abdominal examination, assess uterine contractions and tenderness. A cervical examination is important to assess the effect of labor on the cervix. Inspect the fetal heart rate monitor tracing and uterine tocodynamometry.

C. **Diagnostic Data**
   1. Obtain a **CBC** with **differential** and platelets (and a serum fibrinogen level if the patient is bleeding).
   2. **Urinalysis** (obtained by bladder catheterization) and urine culture and sensitivity are needed.
   3. **Culture the cervix** for *Neisseria* gonorrhea. Obtain a cervical/vaginal/perineal culture and Gram's stain (stat) for group B β-hemolytic-streptococcus.
   4. Perform an **ultrasound** of the fetus to confirm gestational age and to rule out anomalies.
   5. **Consider obtaining an amniocentesis:**
      a. If chorioamnionitis is strongly suspected or if labor does not stop easily with tocolytic agents. (The most common organisms associated with occult intra-amniotic infection in PTL are fusobacteria [25%], bacte-

roides [20%, not *Bacteroides fragilis*], ureaplasma [9%], and *Gardnerella vaginalis* [5%].)

b. In gestations between 32 and 36 weeks, to determine lung maturity.

III. Therapeutic Management

A. Tocolysis

1. **FDA statement on tocolytics.*** The FDA has stated that the use of approved drugs for nonlabeled indications may be entirely appropriate based on medical advances extensively reported in the medical literature:

   The appropriateness or the legality of prescribing approved drugs for uses not included in their official labeling is sometimes a cause of concern and confusion among practitioners. Under the Federal Food, Drug, and Cosmetic (FD&C) Act, a drug approved for marketing may be labeled, promoted, and advertised by the manufacturer only for those uses for which the drug's safety and effectiveness have been established and which the FDA has approved . . .

   The FD&C Act does not, however, limit the manner in which a physician may use an approved drug. Once a product has been approved for marketing, a physician may prescribe it for uses or in treatment regimens or patient populations that are not included in approved labeling. Such "unapproved" or, more precisely, "unlabeled" uses may be appropriate and rational in certain circumstances, and may, in fact, reflect approaches to drug therapy that have been extensively reported in medical literature. . . .

   Before such advances can be added to the approved labeling, however, data substantiating the effectiveness of a new use or regimen must be submitted by the manufacturer to the FDA for evaluation. This may take time and, without the initiative of the drug manufacturer whose product is involved, may never occur. For that reason, accepted medical practice often includes drug use that is not reflected in approved drug labeling.

B. Betamimetic Administration Guidelines

1. **Clinical Criteria**

   a. Betamimetic tocolytics are used for the management of

*From Gabbe SG, Niebyl JR, Simpson JL: *Obstetrics: Normal and Problem Pregnancies*. New York, Churchill Livingstone, 1986. Used by permission.

preterm labor. Fig 15–1 demonstrates the effect of betamimetics at the cellular level. Fig 15–2 demonstrates the chemical structure of epinephrine and β-agonist drugs currently in use in the United States.

b. Table 15–3 summarizes the use of betamimetics and magnesium sulfate for preterm labor.

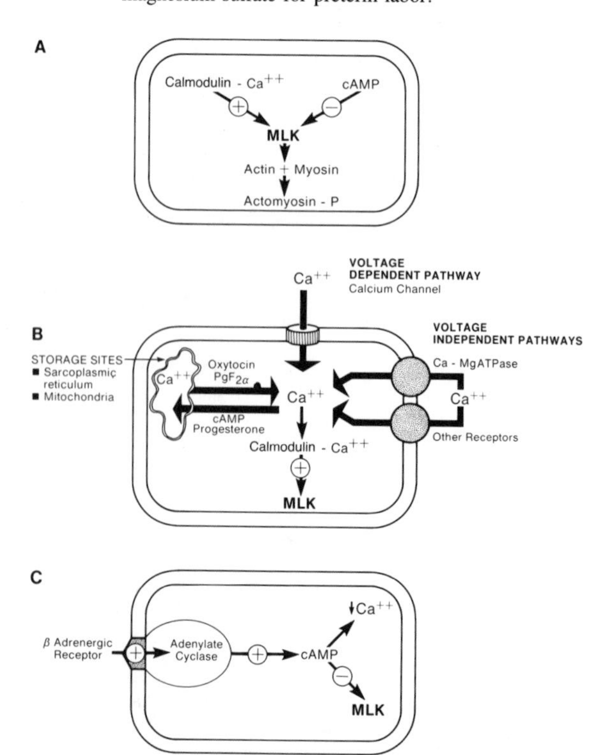

FIG 15–1.

Control of myometrial contractility. Myosin light-chain kinase *(MLK)* is the key enzyme. See text for details. (From Gabbe SG, Niebyl JR, Simpson JL: *Obstetrics: Normal and Problem Pregnancies*. New York, Churchill Livingstone, 1986. Used by permission.)

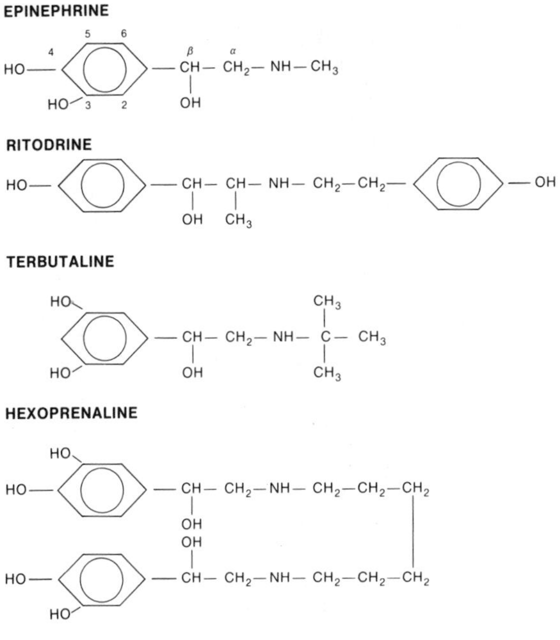

EPINEPHRINE

HO— (ring: 2, 3, 4, 5, 6; HO at 3) —CH(β)(OH)— CH_2(α)— NH— CH_3

RITODRINE

HO— (ring) —CH(OH)— CH(CH_3)— NH— CH_2—CH_2— (ring) —OH

TERBUTALINE

(HO)(HO)(ring) —CH(OH)— CH_2— NH— C(CH_3)(CH_3)— CH_3

HEXOPRENALINE

HO—(HO)(ring) —CH(OH)— CH_2—NH— CH_2—CH_2—CH_2

HO—(HO)(ring) —CH(OH)— CH_2—NH— CH_2—CH_2—CH_2

FIG 15–2.

Structure of epinephrine and β-agonist drugs currently used in the United States. β_2 activity appears to be dependent on large alkyl substitutions on the amino group while maintaining hydroxyl groups at the 3 or 5 position on the benzene ring. (From Gabbe SG, Niebyl JR, Simpson JL: *Obstetrics: Normal and Problem Pregnancies*. New York, Churchill Livingstone, 1986. Used by permission.)

2. **Contraindications**
   a. **Absolute** contraindications to the administration of betamimetic agents are:
      1) Maternal cardiac disease (structural, ischemic, or dysrhythmias)
      2) Eclampsia or preeclampsia
      3) Significant antepartum hemorrhage of any cause
      4) Chorioamnionitis

TABLE 15–3.

Summary of the Use of Betamimetics and Magnesium Sulfate Therapy for Preterm Labor*

Medication	Efficacy	Contraindication†	IV	Doses IM or SC	PO
Ritodrine (Yutopar) (only medication currently approved by FDA for treatment of premature labor)	More effective than placebo or alcohol[1]; as effective as terbutaline in one study[2]	Absolute: severe cardiac disease Use only with extreme caution in: Hyperthyroidism Hypertension Diabetes Anemia Multiple pregnancy Mild cardiac disease	Initial dose: 50–100 μg/min; increase by 50 μg every 10 min until labor stops or unacceptable side effects develop (max dose 350 μg/min); once labor stops maintain IV dose × 12 hr[3]	None currently recommended	10 mg po 30 min prior to stopping IV, then 10 mg po q 2 hr or 20 mg po q 4 hr × 24 hr; if stable may decrease to 10–20 mg q 4–6 hr; max dose 120 mg/day[3]
Terbutaline (Bricanyl, Brethine)	More effective than placebo or alcohol; as effective as ritodrine[2]	Same as above	Initial dose: 10 μg/min; increase by 5 μg/min every 10 min until labor stops or maximum dose of 25 μg/min is reached[4]	250 μg SC 4–6 hr	5 mg q 6–8 hr or 2.5 mg po q 4 hr[4]

Isoxsuprine (Vasodilan)	More effective than placebo; less effective than ritodrine or terbutaline[2]	Same as above	250–500 μg/min starting; slowly increase to 1.0 mg/min if needed[4]	None	5–20 mg po q 3–6 hr[4];
Magnesium sulfate	May be more effective than ethanol[5] and as effective as terbutaline in one study[6]		4 gm loading, then 2 gm/hr until labor stopped	10 gm IM (5 g into each buttock) in addition to 4 g IV; follow with 5 g IM q 4 hr	1 g magnesium gluconate po q 2–4 hr

IM = intramuscularly; IV = intravenously; SC = subcutaneously.

*From Main DM, Main EK: *Obstetrics and Gynecology. A Pocket Reference.* St Louis, Mosby–Year Book, 1984. Used by permission.

†All agents are contraindicated with fetal death in utero, evidence of chorioamnionitis, active vaginal bleeding, eclampsia and severe preeclampsia, and any other obstetric or medical condition that mitigates against prolongation of pregnancy.

1. Merkatz IR, Peter JB, Barden TP: Ritodrine hydrochloride: A betamimetic agent for use in preterm labor. II. Evidence of efficacy. *Obstet Gynecol* 1980; 56:7.
2. Karlsson K, Krantz M, Hamberger L: Comparison of various betamimetics on preterm labor, survival and development of the child, *J Perinat Med* 1980; 8:19.
3. Barden TP, Peter JB, Merkatz IR: Ritodrine hydrochloride: A betamimetic agent for use in preterm labor, I. Pharmacology, clinical history, administration, side effects and safety, *Obstet Gynecol* 1980; 56:1.
4. Barden TP: Premature labor, in Bolognese RJ, Schwartz RH, Schneider J (eds): *Perinatal Medicine, Management of the High Risk Fetus and Neonate* (ed 2). Baltimore, Williams & Wilkins, 1982.
5. Steer CM, Petrie RH: A comparison of magnesium sulfate and alcohol for the prevention of premature labor, *Am J Obstet Gynecol* 1977; 129:1.
6. Miller JM, Keane MWD, Horger EO: A comparison of magnesium sulfate and terbutaline for the arrest of premature labor, a preliminary report, *J Reprod Med* 1982; 27:348.
7. Martin RW, Martin JN Jr, Pryor JA, et al: *Am J Obstet Gynecol* 1988; 158:1440–1445.

5) Fetal mortality or significant abnormality
6) Significant fetal growth retardation
7) Uncontrolled maternal diabetes mellitus
8) Maternal medical conditions that would be seriously affected by the pharmacologic properties of the β-adrenergic agonists, such as hyperthyroidism, uncontrolled hypertension, or hypovolemia
9) Any obstetric or medical condition that contraindicates prolongation of pregnancy

b. Conditions of increased risk and relative contraindications include:
1) Multiple gestation
2) PROM
3) Febrile patient
4) Maternal diabetes (well controlled)
5) Maternal chronic hypertension
6) Patients receiving potassium-depleting diuretics
7) History of severe migraine headaches

C. **Physiologic Effects of β-Adrenergic Stimulation**

1. The **maternal physiologic effects of β_1 and β_2-receptor–mediated stimulation** are detailed in Table 15–4.
2. The **fetal response** is detailed in Table 15–5.

TABLE 15–4.

Physiologic Effects of β-Adrenergic Stimulation*

β_1-Receptor–Mediated	β_2-Receptor–Mediated
Cardiac	Smooth muscle
↑ Heart rate	↓ Uterine activity
↑ Stroke volume	↓ Bronchiolar tone
	↓ Vascular tone
	↓ Intestinal motility
Renal	Renal
↑ Renal blood flow	↑ Renin
	↑ Aldosterone
Metabolic	Metabolic
↑ Lipolysis (↑ ketones)	↑ Insulin
↓ HCO_3	↑ Glycogen release (↑ glucose)
↑ Intracellular K^+	↑ Skeletal muscle lactate

*From Gabbe SG, Niebyl JR, Simpson JL: *Obstetrics: Normal and Problem Pregnancies.* New York, Churchill Livingstone, 1986. Used by permission.

TABLE 15–5.
Fetal Response to β-Adrenergic Receptor Stimulation

Cardiac
↑ Heart rate
Smooth muscle
↓ Vascular tone
Metabolic
↑ Serum glucose during medication administration: subsequent rebound hypoglycemia may occur
↓ Calcium

D. Tocolytic-Related Pulmonary Edema

1. Recommendations to avoid tocolytic-related pulmonary edema during intravenous administration of betamimetics include:
   a. Restrict fluid intake to 2.5 L/day (total IV and oral).
   b. Limit the salt content of fluids; avoid saline and Ringer's lactate solutions.
   c. Restrict the total dose and length of intravenous betamimetic therapy.
   d. Respect contraindications to betamimetic use.
   e. Careful monitoring of patient intake and output.
2. Predisposing factors for pulmonary edema when utilizing betamimetic tocolytic therapy are detailed in Table 15–6.

E. Intravenous Therapy

1. **Ritodrine (Zutopar)**
   a. **Preparation.** Add 150 mg ritodrine (3 ampules) to 500 mL 5% dextrose in water (D_5W) (0.3 mg/mL). The final concentration is such that each 10 mL/hr delivers 50 μg/min.
   b. **Administration**
      1) The initial rate of the infusion is 50–100 μg/min. The rate is increased by increments of 50 μg every 10 minutes until one of the following occurs:
         a) Uterine relaxation
         b) Unacceptable side effects
         c) Maximum rate of 350 μg/min reached
      2) Administer ritodrine according to Table 15–7.
      3) Generally the infusion should be continued for at least 12 hours after uterine contractions cease.

TABLE 15–6.
Pulmonary Edema and Betamimetic Tocolytic Therapy: Predisposing Factors*

Underlying predisposing factors in normal pregnancy
- ↑ Intravascular volume
- ↓ Peripheral vascular resistance
- ↓ Blood viscosity
- ↑ Heart rate
- ↓ Plasma colloid osmotic pressure
- ↑ Pulmonary vascular permeability (?)
- Intrapartum volume shifts

Additive effects of betamimetic therapy
- Further expansion of intravascular volume
- Further ↓ in peripheral vascular resistance
- Further ↓ in blood viscosity
- Further ↑ in heart rate
- Further ↓ in plasma colloid osmotic pressure
- Further ↑ in pulmonary vascular permeability (?)

Extra predisposing medical or treatment factors
- Twins
- Injudicious fluid management
- Heart rate >130 BPM
- Treatment >24 hours
- Unsuspected heart lesions (i.e., mitral stenosis)
- Amnionitis
- Hypertension
- Glucocorticoids (?)

*From Gabbe SG, Niebyl JR, Simpson JL: *Obstetrics: Normal and Problem Pregnancies.* New York, Churchill Livingstone, 1986. Used by permission.

2. **Terbutaline Sulfate**
   a. Preparation
      1) Add 7.5 mg (7.5 ampules) to 500 mL D_5W (0.15 mg/mL).
      2) The final concentration is such that each 10 mL/hr delivers 2.5 μg/min.
   b. Administration
      1) Begin the infusion at 2.5 μg/min.
      2) Increase the infusion by 2.5 μg/min every 20 minutes (to a maximum of 17.5–20 μg/min) until uterine relaxation or marked side effects occur.

TABLE 15–7.
Administration of Ritodrine*

Ritodrine Administration† Concentration: 150 mg/500 mL D5W	
Rate (mL/hr)	Delivers (μg/min)
20	100
30	150
40	200
50	250
60	300
70	350

*From Pharmaceutical Protocol, Long Beach Memorial Medical Center, 1990. Used by permission.
†All infusions must be regulated by an infusion pump.

3) Continue the infusion for at least 12 hours after uterine contractions cease.

3. **Patient Evaluation During Intravenous Therapy**
   a. **Clinical.** Because cardiovascular responses are common and more pronounced during intravenous administration of ritodrine, cardiovascular effects, including the maternal pulse rate, blood pressure, and fetal heart rate, should be closely monitored. Care should be exercised for maternal signs and symptoms of pulmonary edema. Occult cardiac disease may be unmasked with the use of ritodrine or terbutaline.
   b. **Diagnostic Data**
      1) Serum electrolytes, especially potassium, should be monitored during ritodrine therapy
      2) Blood glucose should be monitored during ritodrine or terbutaline therapy in diabetic patients.
   c. **Adverse reactions** to ritodrine and terbutaline include alterations in maternal blood pressure, tachycardia, a transient elevation of blood sugar and insulin levels, a reduction in serum potassium, tremor, nausea, vomiting, headache, erythema, nervousness, restlessness, emotional upset, and anxiety. The severity of the

symptoms may determine if the medications should be discontinued.

F. Oral Therapy

1. **Ritrodrine or Terbutaline**
   a. Give one tablet (ritodrine 10 mg or terbutaline 2.5 mg) approximately 30 minutes before the termination of intravenous tocolytic therapy.
      1) The usual dosage schedule for oral maintenance is one tablet every 2 hours, if tolerated.
      2) The total daily dose of ritodrine or terbutaline should not exceed 120 mg of ritodrine or 30 mg of terbutaline.
   b. Night doses should be held unless the patient awakens. If she does wake up during the night,
      1) Check her pulse.
      2) A dose may be given if the criteria for the pulse rate are met and it has been at least 2 hours since the previous dose was given.
2. **Patient Evaluation During Oral Tocolytic Therapy**
   a. Check her pulse before each dose is given. Subsequent doses should be given only if her pulse is at or below 115 beats/min.
      1) If her pulse exceeds 115 beats/min, recheck it in 30 to 60 minutes. Administer the dose when her pulse rate drops to 115 beats/min or less.
      2) A new dosing schedule should be initiated at any time doses are held.
      3) If it becomes necessary to hold two or more consecutive doses, the physician should be notified.
   b. If continued therapy is required on an outpatient basis, the patient should be instructed how to take her pulse. Discuss a course of action with her in the event that her pulse rate exceeds 115 beats/min.

G. Subcutaneous Infusion of Terbutaline

1. **Benefits Over Oral Terbutaline.** Subcutaneous dosing minimizes the total terbutaline dose required, with subsequent reduction of side effects and tachyphylaxis.
2. **Administration**
   a. Dosing may be started at a basal rate of 0.05 mL/hour.
   b. Boluses of medication may be scheduled for periods of peak uterine activity.

3. Consult your local subcutaneous pump specialist if this route of administration is desired.
4. The cost of this method of medication administration is much greater than with oral tablets.

H. Magnesium Sulfate Tocolysis

1. **Contraindications to tocolysis** (Table 15–8).
2. **Mechanism of Action.** The exact mechanism by which magnesium sulfate ($MgSO_4$) reduces uterine activity remains an enigma. The theory that has the most support is that $MgSO_4$ competes with calcium at either the motor end plate, thus reducing excitation of the muscle, or the cellular membrane, where depolarization occurs.
3. **Administration**
   a. Only **intravenous** administration of $MgSO_4$ achieves a steady elevation of serum magnesium levels.
      1) **Loading Dose:** Dose of 4–6 g administered during a period of 20 minutes
      2) **Maintenance Dosage:** Dosage of 2–3 g/hr titrated according to the patient's deep tendon reflexes (DTRs) and serum magnesium level (The dosage may be reduced after uterine quiescence.)
      3) **Sample Orders**
         a) 50 g $MgSO_4$ in 1 L dextrose 5% Ringer's lactate (D5LR)
         b) Infuse 4 g (80 mL) over a period of 20 minutes (loading dose)
         c) Then 2 g/hr (40 mL/hr)
         d) Fluid restrict to 100 mL/hr (total intake)
         e) IV—Ringer's lactate alternate with D5LR at rate appropriate for fluid restriction

TABLE 15–8.

Contraindications to Tocolysis

Contraindications to Tocolysis
Cervical dilatation >4 cm
Ruptured membranes
Intrauterine infection
Severe intrauterine growth retardation
Clinically significant bleeding
Fetal anomalies incompatible with life

f) Nothing by mouth except ice chips
g) Strict monitoring of input and output
h) In-and-out catheterization or Foley catheterization placement prn
i) Mg^{++} level 2 hours after load; then every 4 hours

b. **Intramuscular** administration may be utilized when the continuous intravenous route is not possible.
1) **Loading Dose.** Administer 5 g in a 50% solution (equally with dextrose in water) in each buttock (a total of 10 g) in addition to 4 g in 250 mL 5% dextrose in water infused intravenously during a period of 20 minutes.
2) **Maintenance Dose.** Administer 5 g in a 50% solution every 4 hours. Before administration, examine deep tendon reflexes, respiratory rates, and urine output.

c. **Oral Magnesium Gluconate**
1) Administer 1 g oral magnesium gluconate (54 mg elemental magnesium) every 2–4 hours.
2) A preliminary study by Martin et al. suggests that this therapy may be as effective an oral tocolytic as β-agonists.

4. **Patient Evaluation During Intravenous Therapy**
a. **Adverse reactions** may include nausea, flushing, drowsiness, blurred vision, chest discomfort, and difficulty breathing (Table 15–9).
b. Evaluate the patient approximately 2 hours after the loading dose is given and then every 4–6 hours depending on the patient's status and magnesium infusion rate (Table 15–10).
c. In case of **magnesium sulfate** toxicity, administer 1 g **calcium gluconate** intravenously by slow push over 3 minutes.
d. A clinical evaluation of the patient should be performed every hour.
1) Respirations
a) Maintain at a minimum of 12 per minute.
b) A diminished respiratory rate may indicate pulmonary edema.
c) If respirations are depressed, consider discontinuing magnesium therapy.

TABLE 15–9.

Maternal and Fetal Side Effects of Magnesium Sulfate*

	Maternal	Fetal/Neonatal
Magnesium sulfate		
Metabolic	↑ Serum magnesium ↓ Calcium—usually within lower limits of normal; after administration for several days may become symptomaticly low[2] ↑ Parathyroid hormone[1] No change in calcitonin or phosphorus[1]	↑ Serum magnesium[1] ↓ Serum calcium[1] No change in PTH or calcitonin[1]
Cardiovascular	Transient decrease in systolic and diastolic BP[3] ↓ Respiratory rate[3] No change in pulse or temperature[3] Slight increase in uterine blood flow in sheep[4]	No change in fetal heart rate[3]
Pulmonary	Pulmonary edema reported in two cases also treated with corticosteroids[5]	
Toxic	Cardiac arrest Respiratory arrest NOTE: Absent patellar reflexes may represent impending toxicity rather than therapeutic level; need to monitor serum magnesium levels[6]	

Selected references:

1. Cruikshank DP, et al: Effects of magnesium sulfate treatment on perinatal calcium metabolism, *Am J Obstet Gynecol* 1979; 134:243.
2. Eisenbud E, LoBue CC: Hypocalcemia after therapeutic use of magnesium sulfate, *Arch Intern Med* 1976; 136:688.
3. Young BK, Weinstein HM: Effects of magnesium sulfate on toxemic patients in labor, *Obstet Gynecol* 1977; 49:681.
4. Dandavino A, et al: Circulatory effects of magnesium sulfate in normotensive and renal hypertensive pregnant sheep, *Am J Obstet Gynecol* 1977; 127:769.
5. Elliott JP, et al: Pulmonary edema associated with magnesium sulfate and betamethasone administration, *Am J Obstet Gynecol* 1979; 134:717.
6. Sibai BM, et al: Reassessment of intravenous $MgSO_4$ therapy in preeclampsia-eclampsia, *Obstet Gynecol* 1981; 57:199.

*From Main DM, Main EK: *Obstetrics and Gynecology. A Pocket Reference.* St Louis, Mosby–Year Book, 1984. Used by permission.

TABLE 15–10.
Effect of Magnesium Sulfate Therapy

Magnesium Level	Physiologic Effect
4–7 mEq/L (5–8 mg/dL)	Therapeutic range
8–10 mEq/L (9–12 mg/dL)	Loss of deep tendon reflexes
13–15 mEq/L (16–18 mg/dL)	Respiratory arrest
15–20 mEq/L (18—25 mg/dL)	Heart block, cardiac conduction defects (peaked T waves, prolonged PR and QRS intervals)
20–25 mEq/L (25–30 mg/dL)	Cardiac arrest

2) Urine output (U/O)
   a) U/O should be at least 30 mL/hour.
   b) A decreased U/O may result in a high serum magnesium level.
3) DTRs should be present.
4) Obtain a serum magnesium level if DTRs are lost, the respiratory rate decreases, or the U/O diminishes below 30 mL/hr.

e. **Diagnostic Data**
   1) Evaluate the serum creatinine level upon initiation of magnesium tocolysis (because magnesium is excreted by the kidneys).
   2) Consider obtaining a serum magnesium level 2 hr after loading dose then every 4–6 hr depending on the patient's status.

I. Tocolysis, Miscellaneous Medications

1. **Indomethacin**
   a. **Mechanism of Action.** Indomethacin acts by inhibiting prostaglandin synthesis at the cyclooxygenase enzyme. Prostaglandins are part of the final pathway of smooth muscle contraction.
   b. **Indication.** Because of the serious fetal side effects, indomethacin should be utilized only with very immature gestations in which standard tocolysis failed. Recent evidence suggests that indomethacin not be used for at more than 48 hours.
   c. **Contraindications**
      1) Maternal

a) Peptic ulcer disease
b) History of salicylate sensitivity

2) Obstetric
a) See Table 15–8.
b) Oligohydramnios.

d. **Administration**

1) **Loading Dose**
a) Premedicate the patient with 1 g sucralfate (Carafate) 30 minutes before all oral doses of indomethacin.
b) Administer 50 mg orally or rectally by suppository.

2) **Maintenance dosing** is accomplished by administering 25 mg orally every 4 hours, preceded 30 minutes earlier by Carafate.

3) The **duration of therapy** is usually only 24 hours. If contractions have not subsided by this time, a second course of indomethacin may be given.

e. **Patient Evaluation**

1) **Diagnostic Data.** A fetal ultrasound must be performed before administration of this medication to assure that the amniotic fluid volume is sufficient.

2) **Adverse reactions** include:
a) Oligohydramnios
b) Intrauterine closure of the ductus arteriosus (not described in fetuses treated for less than 48 hours)
c) Neonatal pulmonary hypertension (not described in fetuses treated for less than 48 hours)

2. **Calcium Channel Blockers (Nifedipine)**

a. **Mechanism of Action.** Calcium channel blockers prevent calcium entry into the cell, thus inhibiting smooth muscle contraction. Nifedipine is a long-acting vasodilator.

b. **Contraindications**

1) See Table 15–8.
2) Sick-sinus syndrome.
3) Second or third degree atrioventricular block.
4) Shock.
5) Congestive heart failure.

c. **Administration**
   1) Ten to 20 mg orally every 8 hours; this may be increased to a maximum of 10 mg orally every 3 hours.
   2) Ninety percent of the medication is absorbed when ingested orally or sublingually.

d. The **onset of action** is 20 minutes when ingested orally (with a peak effect in 1–2 hours) and 3 minutes when taken sublingually (peak effect in 10 minutes).

e. The initial **half-life** is 2.5–3.0 hours.

f. **Adverse reactions** are uncommon, occurring in less than 10% of patients.
   1) Fatigue
   2) Headache
   3) Dizziness
   4) Skin rash
   5) Peripheral edema

g. If the patient is taking **digoxin** concurrently, its serum level may rise.

3. **Diazoxide**

   a. **Mechanism of Action.** Diazoxide is thought to activate adenylate cyclase, which reduces the concentration of intracellular calcium by extruding it from the cell, thus decreasing systemic vascular resistance. Diazoxide is metabolized in the liver; however 50% is excreted by the kidneys in its original form.

   b. **Contraindications**
      1) See Table 15–3.
      2) Hypovolemia.

   c. **Administration**
      1) Give 5 mg/kg (average dose 300 mg) intravenously over 15–20 minutes.
      2) Cease administration of the medication if the patient develops any cardiovascular symptoms.
      3) A second dose may be given if labor recurs.

   d. **Patient Evaluation**
      1) Clinical evaluation. Evaluate the patient's vital signs (especially heart rate and blood pressure) frequently.
      2) Adverse reactions
         a) Hypotension
         b) If administered too rapidly, your patient may complain of dizziness, nausea, and headache.

J. Regarding the vaginal/introital/perineal **Gram's stain and culture** for group B β-streptococcus:

1. In place of Gram's stain, consider a rapid test or treat all patients until culture results return.
2. If the Gram's stain shows gram-positive cocci in pairs, initiate treatment with **ampicillin,** 500 mg orally every 6 hours (or erythromycin, 500 mg orally every 6 hours, if the patient is allergic to penicillin).
3. If the culture fails to grow group B β-streptococcus after initiating treatment on the basis of Gram's stain findings, discontinue ampicillin.
4. If the culture grows group B β-streptococcus, or if the patient has a history of a positive culture for group B strep that was treated, continue ampicillin, 500 mg (erythromycin if penicillin allergic), orally every 6 hours for 10 days. If the patient goes into **active labor,** treat her with **IV ampicillin** (erythromycin if penicillin allergic). Obtain another vaginal specimen for culture after treatment is completed.
5. **If the cervical culture is positive for gonorrhea,** treat per recommendations from the Centers for Disease Control (see Appendix Q) and subsequently reculture.
6. Consider using steroids to accelerate fetal lung maturity (see Appendix M).

K. Before transfer to the floor and discharge from the hospital, the patient will have undergone tocolysis and may be on an oral tocolytic agent (i.e., terbutaline).

L. While on the antepartum floor, she is assessed daily. As her disease becomes more stable, her activity is liberalized.

1. **First Day.** Strict bed rest is usually prescribed. She is to have 60 minutes of uterine monitoring twice daily throughout the remainder of hospitalization. If five or more contractions per hour are present, the patient requires further evaluation or treatment (or both).
2. **Second Day.** The patient is given bathroom privileges only. If rare or no uterine contractions occur, the patient's condition is assessed to be stable.
3. **When the patient is discharged,** give her a prescription for her tocolytic agent. Patients with greater cervical dilation are usually observed for a day or two longer than those with minimal cervical change.

M. **Weekly office visits** with cervical examinations are recommended. In the presence of recurring uterine contractions or further cervical change, send the patient to labor and delivery for monitoring and care.

N. **Consider** home uterine contraction monitoring with daily nurse contact.

BIBLIOGRAPHY

Adamsons K, Wallach RC: Treating preterm labor with diazoxide. *Contemp Obstet Gynecol (Interview)*, pp 161–177, January 1988.

Berkowitz RL, Coustan DR, Mochizuki TK: *Handbook for Prescribing Medications During Pregnancy*. Boston, Little, Brown, 1986.

Cartis SN, Toig G, Heddinger LA, et al: A double-blind study comparing ritodrine and terbutaline in the treatment of preterm labor. *Am J Obstet Gynecol* 1984; 150:7.

De Wit W, Van Mourik I, Wiesenhaan PF: Prolonged maternal indomethacin therapy associated with oligohydramnios. Case reports. *Br J Obstet Gynaecol* 1988; 95:303–305.

Ferguson JE II, Schutz T, Pershe R, et al: Nifedipine pharmacokinetics during preterm labor tocolysis. *Am J Obstet Gynecol* 1989; 161:1485–1490.

Gabbe SG, Niebyl JR, Simpson JL: *Obstetrics: Normal and Problem Pregnancies*. New York, Churchill Livingstone, 1986.

Hatjis CG, Swain M: Systemic tocolysis for premature labor is associated with an increased incidence of pulmonary edema in the presence of maternal infection. *Am J Obstet Gynecol* 1988; 159:723–728.

King JF, Grant A, Keirse MJNC, et al: Beta-mimetics in preterm labour: An overview of the randomized controlled trials. *Br J Obstet Gynaecol* 1988; 95:211–222.

Lam F: The scientific rationale for low-dose terbutaline pump therapy in the management of premature labor. Is β2-adrenoceptor desensitization by down regulation the cause of tocolytic breakthrough? (Unpublished manuscript. Author is at Children's Hospital of San Francisco. Date unknown.)

Lam F, Gill PJ, Smith M, et al: Use of subcutaneous terbutaline pump for long-term tocolysis. (Abstract presented at University of California at Irvine in 1988.)

Main DM, Main EK: *Obstetrics and Gynecology. A Pocket Reference*. St Louis, Mosby–Year Book, 1984.

Mamelle N, Munoz F: Occupational working conditions and preterm birth: A reliable scoring system. *Am J Epidemiol* 1987; 126:150–152.

Martin RW, Martin JN Jr, Pryor JA, et al: *Am J Obstet Gynecol* 1988; 158:1440–1445.

Moise KJ Jr, Huhta JC, Sharif DS, et al: Indomethacin in the treatment of preterm labor. *N Engl J Med* 1988; 319:327–331.

Moore BR, Briggs GG, Freeman RK: Terbutaline for tocolysis: Do advantages outweigh risks? *Contemp Obstet Gynecol,* September 1988.

Niebyl J: Indomethacin for preterm labor (Interview). *Contemp Obstet Gynecol* 1988; 69–72.

Niebyl JR, Johnson JWC: Inhibition of preterm labor. *Clin Obstet Gynecol* 1980; 23:115.

Niebyl JR, Witter FR: Neonatal outcome after indomethacin treatment for preterm labor. *Am J Obstet Gynecol* 1986; 155:747–749.

Polowczyk D, Tejani N, Lauersen N, et al: Evaluation of seven- to nine-year-old children exposed to ritodrine in utero. *Obstet Gynecol* 1984; 64:485–488.

Porto M: Home uterine activity monitoring: Essential tool or expensive accessory? *Contemp Obstet Gynecol* 1990; 35:114–123.

Romero R, Mazor M, Oyarzun E: Role of intra-amniotic infection in preterm labor. *Contemp Obstet Gynecol,* December 1988; 94–106.

Stubblefield PG, Heyl PS: Treatment of premature labor with subcutaneous terbutaline. *Obstet Gynecol* 1982; 59:457.

Wilkins I, Lynch L, Mehalek KE, et al: Efficacy and side effects of magnesium sulfate and ritodrine as tocolytic agents. *Am J Obstet Gynecol* 1988; 159:685–689.

Zatuchni GI, Slupik RI: *Obstetrics and Gynecology Drug Handbook.* St.Louis, Mosby–Year Book, 1991.

PREGNANCY-INDUCED HYPERTENSION/ PREECLAMPSIA

16

I. Background

A. Definitions

1. **Mild Pregnancy-Induced Hypertension (PIH).** BP >140/90 mm Hg (or a 30 mm Hg rise in systolic BP, or a 15 mm Hg rise in diastolic BP measured on two occasions, 6 hours apart) or a mean arterial BP of 105 mm Hg (or an increase of 20 mm Hg), occurring for the first time during pregnancy
2. **Mild Preeclampsia.** PIH Plus **proteinuria, edema, or both**
   a. **Proteinuria** is the excretion of ≥0.3 g of protein per liter of urine in a 24-hour specimen or 0.1 g/L in a random specimen.
   b. **Edema** is diagnosed by:
      1) Clinically evident swelling, nonresponsive to 12 hours of bed rest, or
      2) A weight gain of 5 pounds or more in the preceding week
3. **Severe preeclampsia** is the presence of a BP of 160/110 (on two occasions, 6 hours apart, with the patient at bed rest on her left side) in addition to any of the following, occurring for the first time during pregnancy:
   a. **Proteinuria** of ≥5 g in 24 hours (or 3–4+ on a qualitative examination)
   b. **Oliguria** (≤500 mL/24 hr)
   c. **Cerebral** or **visual disturbances**

d. **Epigastric pain**
e. **HELLP syndrome** (hemolysis, elevated liver enzymes, and low platelet count)
f. **Pulmonary edema** or cyanosis

4. **Eclampsia** is the occurrence of seizures in a preeclamptic patient that cannot be attributed to other causes.
5. The term **PIH** will be used throughout the remainder of this chapter to refer to PIH and its related disorders (preeclampsia and eclampsia).

B. Incidence

1. PIH occurs in 5% of pregnancies.
2. It is more frequent in primigravidas and in patients in lower socioeconomic groups.
3. The prevalence of PIH increases near term and the disease usually resolves by 6 weeks' postpartum.

C. Etiology. The exact cause of PIH is unknown, but theories include uteroplacental ischemia, disseminated intravascular coagulation, poor nutrition, and immunologic disturbances.

D. Risk factors for **PIH** include:

1. Multiple gestation
2. Hydramnios
3. Diabetes mellitus
4. Prior history of chronic hypertension (HTN) (25%–30% of patients with chronic HTN go on to develop PIH)
5. Family history of PIH
6. Vascular disease
7. Hydatidiform mole (The onset of PIH in the second trimester suggests this cause.)

E. Perinatal Morbidity and Mortality

1. Abruptio placentae, which is increased in preeclamptic and eclamptic patients, results in a perinatal mortality rate of 460/1,000.
2. Prematurity, intrauterine growth retardation, and hypoxic episodes during eclamptic seizures also place the fetus at greater risk of morbidity and mortality.

F. Maternal Morbidity and Mortality

1. PIH is considered one of the leading causes of maternal morbidity.
2. Mothers with preeclampsia are at increased risk for:
   a. Placental abruption
   b. Vascular damage to all their organ systems
   c. Thrombocytopenia
   d. Disseminated intravascular coagulation

3. The mortality rate in patients with preeclampsia is unchanged from that seen in patients with uncomplicated pregnancies; however, it is increased in patients with eclampsia.

II. Evaluation

A. **History.** Inquire about the presence of risk factors for PIH, i.e., diabetes mellitus, previous chronic hypertension, and vascular disease. Ask the patient if she has noticed swelling of her face and extremities (i.e., are your rings or shoes [or both] tighter?) and inquire about neurologic signs (i.e., headaches, tinnitus).

B. **Physical Examination.** Perform a complete physical examination. Measure the patient's BP (with the correct size cuff) yourself, with the patient in a left lateral decubitus position and the cuff on the superior portion of the arm. In patients with possible **PIH,** be sure to examine for face, hand, and pretibial edema. A funduscopic examination is important for evidence of chronic **HTN.** Palpate the abdomen for any tenderness or pain.

C. **Diagnostic Data**
   1. Obtain a **urinalysis.** (First examine the urine dipstick in the ER. If $\geq$1+ protein is present, send a specimen obtained by bladder catheterization to the laboratory for evaluation.) Proteinuria indicates renal involvement.
   2. Send a **CBC with platelet count** (an elevated hemoglobin and hematocrit indicate hemoconcentration; thrombocytopenia indicates platelet consumption).
   3. An **AST** (SGOT) or **ALT** (SGPT), or both, will identify hepatic involvement.
   4. **Uric acid, creatinine,** and **BUN** will indicate the degree of renal involvement.
   5. Consider obtaining a **24-hour urine collection** for protein and creatinine to examine renal function (calculate the creatinine clearance) and proteinuria (>300 mg/24 hr is significant).

III. Therapeutic Management (Fig 16–1)

A. **Severe preeclampsia** and **eclampsia** warrant immediate delivery regardless of gestational age.
   1. **Seizure prophylaxis**
      a. **$MgSO_4$** is commonly used in the United States to pre-

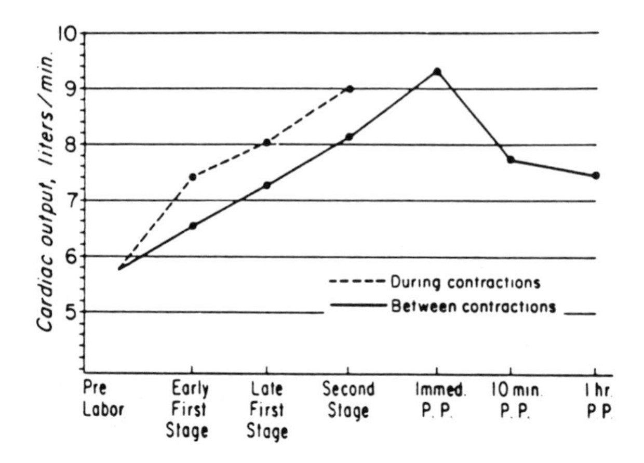

FIG 16–1.
Management of preeclampsia and eclampsia.

vent eclamptic seizures. Initiate $MgSO_4$ therapy with a 4 g load over 20 min followed by 2 g/hr. Please refer to Chapter 15 for details of $MgSO_4$ side effects and patient management guidelines.

b. **Dilantin** is commonly used in other countries as eclamptic seizure prophylaxis.
   1) The **loading dose** is based on the patient's weight (10 mg/kg). Dilantin may be diluted in normal saline, and piggybacked into the mainline IV. Run at a rate no greater than 50 mg/min.
   2) A **second bolus** (5 mg/kg) is given 2 hr after the load.
   3) **Dilantin levels** need to be checked approximately 6 hr and 12 hr after the second bolus (therapeutic range 10–20 ug/ml; to be routinely drawn immediately before a scheduled dose is given). The measured Dilantin level represents the combined bound and unbound fractions of dilantin, whereas the therapeutic effect of this drug is based on only the unbound portion (usually 10%). When serum albumin is low, the unbound fraction of dilantin is cor-

3) **Dilantin levels** need to be checked approximately 6 hr and 12 hr after the second bolus (therapeutic range 10–20 ug/ml; to be routinely drawn immediately before a scheduled dose is given). The measured Dilantin level represents the combined bound and unbound fractions of dilantin, whereas the therapeutic effect of this drug is based on only the unbound portion (usually 10%). When serum albumin is low, the unbound fraction of dilantin is correspondingly increased. To correct for a low albumin level, use the formula:

$$C_{normal} = \frac{C\ \text{observed}}{0.9 \times (\text{albumin concentration}) + 0.1}$$

C_{normal} = dilantin concentration that would have been observed had the patient's albumin concentration been normal.

$C_{observed}$ = measured dilantin concentration

This equation assumes that the unbound fraction is 0.1 when the albumin is normal.

4) **Maintenance doses** are administered initially 12 hr after the second bolus, then every 8–12 hr based on serum levels. The dose is 200 mg po or IV, and is to be continued for 3–5 days.
5) **Adverse reactions** include
   a) Bradycardia and heart block.
   b) Ataxia, slurred speech, nystagmus, mental confusion, decreased coordination.
   c) Nausea, vomiting, constipation.
   d) Local irritation, inflammation, and tenderness at the injection site.

2. Use continuous fetal and uterine monitoring.
3. Consider placement of a central line for fluid management (Tables 16–1 and 16–2).
4. Place a Foley catheter for accurate measurement of urine output.
5. Induce delivery if the patient is not in labor and no fetal or maternal indications for an operative delivery are present.
6. Administer **hydralazine** (Apresoline) in a dose of 2.5 mg intravenous push (IVP) (slowly) if the diastolic BP is persistently >105–110. The patient may require additional

TABLE 16–1.
Normal Resting Hemodynamic Values*, †

	Non-pregnant	Pregnant
Pressure measurements		
Central venous (M) (superior vena cava)	1–10 mm Hg	No change
Right atrium (M)	0–8 mm Hg	No change
Right ventricle (Sys.)	15–30 mm Hg	No sig. change‡
(E.D.)	0–8 mm Hg	"
Pulmonary artery (Sys.)	15–30 mm Hg	No sig. change‡
(E.D.)	3–12 mm Hg	"
(M)	9–16 mm Hg	"
Pulmonary artery wedge (M) (and left atrium)	3–10 mm Hg	No sig. change‡
Left ventricle (Sys.)	100–140 mm Hg	No sig. change‡
(E.D.)	3–12 mm Hg	"
Flow and resistances		
Cardiac output	4.0–7.0 L/min	↑ 30%–45%
Cardiac index	2.8–4.2 L/min/m^2	↑ 30%–45%
Total systemic resistance	770–1500 dyn-s/cm^3	↓ ~25%
Pulmonary vascular resistance	20–120 dyn-s/cm^3	↓ ~25%

*From Main DM, Main EK: *Obstetrics and Gynecology. A Pocket Reference.* St Louis, Mosby–Year Book, 1984. Used by permission.
†Normal Non-pregnant Data, in Barry WH, Grossman W: Cardiac catheterization, in Braunwald E (ed). *Heart Disease: A Textbook of Cardiovascular Medicine, vol 1.* Philadelphia, WB Saunders, 1980, p 289.
‡While normal ranges have not been established by formal studies, available data indicate these values are not significantly changed by pregnancy.
Note: M = Mean, Sys = Systolic, and E.D. = End Diastolic.

doses (the dose may be repeated after 5–10 minutes if her BP does not decrease). Hydralazine requires 20 minutes for its full effect to be manifested. Aim for a diastolic BP >90 mm Hg. If her diastolic BP decreases further than this, uteroplacental insufficiency may occur.

B. Long-term Antepartum Care

1. Preterm patients with mild disease are kept on bed rest (with bathroom privileges) in the hospital, preferably in the left lateral decubitus position. After diagnosis, patients undergo antepartum monitoring until delivery. Consider performing an amniocentesis near term to assess fetal lung

TABLE 16–2.
Pulmonary Artery Wedge Pressures*

Aliases: Pulmonary wedge pressure, pulmonary capillary wedge pressure, and pulmonary artery occlusion pressure.

Provides information on: (1) level of pulmonary venous pressure which is a major determinate of pulmonary congestion; (2) left ventricular filling pressure which allows estimation of cardiac performance. Therefore, wedge pressures can predict pulmonary edema with reasonable accuracy *given normal colloid osmotic pressure and normal pulmonary vascular permeability.*

Advantages over central venous pressure monitoring:

1. More complete cardiovascular information.
2. CVP inaccurately monitors cardiac performance in patients with myocardial infarction, peritonitis, ischemic ST-T EKG changes, other cardio-respiratory diseases, and severe preeclampsia.

Suggested indications in Ob/Gyn:

1. Surgery and/or labor and delivery of a patient with New York Heart Association Class 3 or 4 cardiac disease.
2. Aortic outflow tract obstruction during delivery.
3. Hypovolemic shock secondary to severe intrapartum blood loss or severe postpartum hemorrhage not responsive to initial fluid therapy.
4. Septic shock requiring volume resuscitation or the use of vasopressor agents.
5. Severe preeclampsia and eclampsia complicated by oliguria, pulmonary edema, or hypovolemia secondary to hemorrhage.
6. Suspected amniotic fluid embolus with vascular collapse.
7. Cardiac failure with suspected pulmonary edema.
8. Intraoperative and postoperative monitoring of fluid therapy in gynecologic oncology patients undergoing radical surgery.

General references: Cotton DB, Benedetti TJ: Use of the Swan-Ganz catheter in obstetrics and gynecology. *Obstet Gynecol* 1980; 56:641, and Pace NL: A critique of flow-directed pulmonary arterial catheterization, *Anesthesiology* 1977; 47:455.

*From Main DM, Main EK: *Obstetrics and Gynecology. A Pocket Reference.* St Louis, Mosby–Year Book, 1984. Used by permission.

maturity. Plan the delivery according to the results of lung maturity testing.

2. In addition to the preceding, the patient's orders for the floor should include:
   a. BP monitoring every 4 hours during the day
   b. Evaluation of patellar reflexes daily
   c. Record of daily weight
   d. Dipstick of urine every morning for protein
   e. CBC, creatinine, and AST (SGOT) twice weekly

f. Fetal movement counts to be performed by the patient (provide instruction)
g. Notify physician of any patient complaints of:
   1) Persistent occipital headache
   2) Visual symptoms
   3) Epigastric pain

3. These patients are usually admitted to the hospital for the duration of their pregnancy. If the **PIH** worsens, consider delivery. For persistent diastolic BP's greater than 105, consider administration of hydralazine in addition to delivery.
4. Consider weekly administration of steroids to facilitate fetal surfactant production.

BIBLIOGRAPHY

Dommisse J: Phenytoin sodium and magnesium sulfate in the management of eclampsia. *Br J Obstet Gynecol* 1990; 97:104–109.

Friedman SA: Preeclampsia: A review of the role of prostaglandins. *Obstet Gynecol* 1988; 71:122–137.

Klonoff-Cohen HS, Savitz DA, Cefalo RC, et al: An epidemiologic study of contraception and preeclampsia. *JAMA* 1989; 262:3143–3147.

Ryan G, Lange IR, Naugler MA: Clinical experience with phenytoin prophylaxis in severe preeclampsia. *Am J Obstet Gynecol* 1989; 16:1297–1304.

Sibai BM: Definitive therapy for pregnancy induced hypertension. *Contemp Obstet Gynecol* 1988; pp 51–66, May.

Sibai BM: Preeclampsia-eclampsia: Maternal and perinatal outcomes. *Contemp Obstet Gynecol,* 1988; pp 109–118, December.

Spitz B, Magness RR, Cox SM, et al: Low dose aspirin. I. Effect on angiotensin II pressor responses and blood prostaglandin concentrations in pregnant women sensitive to angiotensin II. *Am J Obstet Gynecol* 1988; 159:1035–1043.

Wallenburg HCS, Makovitz JW, Dekker GA, et al: Low dose aspirin prevents pregnancy-induced hypertension and preeclampsia in angiotensin-sensitive primigravidae. *Lancet* 1986; pp 1–3, Jan 4.

Weinstein L: Syndrome of hemolysis, elevated liver enzymes, and low platelet count: A severe consequence of hypertension in pregnancy. *Am J Obstet Gynecol* 1982; 142:159.

ANTEPARTUM HEMORRHAGE 17

I. Background

A. **Incidence.** Antepartum bleeding occurs in 3.8% of pregnancies that progress beyond 20 weeks' gestation.

B. **Etiology.** The most common causes are **abruptio placentae, placenta previa,** and **vasa previa.** Other causes of third trimester bleeding, which most likely represent <1% of all bleeding cases, include:
   1. Cervicitis
   2. Cervical erosions
   3. Endocervical polyps
   4. Cancer of the cervix
   5. Vaginal, vulvar, and cervical varicosities
   6. Vaginal infections
   7. Foreign bodies
   8. Bloody show
   9. Degenerating uterine fibroids

C. **Perinatal Morbidity and Mortality**
   1. First and early second trimester bleeding is an indicator of total placenta previa and a decreased chance of carrying the fetus near term.
   2. Modern obstetric care and neonatal intensive care units have led to a marked decrease in maternal mortality and an improvement in fetal outcome.
   3. The most frequent cause for an indicated delivery is bleeding.
   4. Perinatal mortality:
      a. Placenta previa 8%–11%
      b. Abruptio placentae 15%
      c. Vasa previa >50%

II. Hemorrhage Assessment

A. Classification (Table 17–1)

B. Physiology

1. Pregnant patients usually do not demonstrate the expected early signs of **volume depletion.** This is the result of the 40% blood volume expansion achieved by 30 weeks' gestation. Thus **it is difficult for the practitioner to adequately assess the blood volume deficit** in these patients.
2. The **physiologic response** to bleeding occurs in two phases. Acutely, vasoconstriction occurs to maintain essential organ flow. Chronically (results not manifest for at least the first 4 hours after the bleeding episode) transcapillary refill may replace up to 30% of the lost volume.

C. Hemoglobin and hematocrit (Hb; Hct) are frequently used to assess the volume loss.

1. Because effects of transcapillary refill are not manifest for at least the first 4 hours after acute bleeding, no significant change is seen in these values during this time unless the patient has bled severely.
2. The infusion of IV fluids may result in an earlier lowering of the measured hemoglobin/hematocrit level.

TABLE 17–1.
Classification of Obstetric Hemorrhage

	Bleeding		
Clinical Signs	Mild	Moderate	Severe*
Vital signs	Within normal limits	Elevated pulse Orthostatic BP Tachypnea	Tachycardia Unrecordable BP Tachypnea
Evidence of circulation volume deficit	None	Subtle perfusion changes (delayed refilling of hypothenar area when squeezed)	Cold, clammy skin Fetal distress or death
Urine output	Within normal limits	Possibly decreased	Oliguria/anuria
Intravascular volume lost	<15%	20%–25%	>30%

*When a woman loses more than 40% of her blood volume, she will be in profound shock. Circulatory collapse and cardiac arrest will occur if volume resuscitation is not begun immediately.

D. **Urine output** (U/O) will usually decrease before any other signs of decreased perfusion are manifest.

1. Renal blood flow is closely correlated with urine production. If a patient is producing at least 30 mL of urine an hour, she is euvolemic.
2. If she produces less than 30 mL of urine per hour after an acute bleeding episode, she requires volume replacement and careful monitoring of her fluid status.

III. Abruptio Placentae

A. **Definition.** Abruptio placentae is the premature separation of a normally implanted placenta. Different classes of abruption are defined by the size of the retroplacental blood clot at delivery or by the clinical setting. A **marginal sinus rupture** is an abruption limited to the margin of the placenta.

B. **Incidence**

1. This disorder occurs in 1%–3% of deliveries and accounts for two thirds of antepartum hemorrhages.
2. The incidence of abruptio placentae increases as term approaches.
3. More than 90% of infants involved weigh more than 1,500 g at delivery.
4. Twenty percent of patients manifest the condition before 28 weeks' gestation, 20% between 28 and 33 weeks, and 22%–40% between 32 and 36 weeks.

C. **Etiology.** The primary cause is unknown, but the factors related to abruptio placentae include:

1. **Maternal Hypertension** and/or **Vascular Disease.** These are responsible for up to 50% of fatal fetal/neonatal cases.
2. **High Parity.** The incidence of abruptio placentae is 1% in primiparas and 2.5% in grand multiparas.
3. **Poor Nutrition,** especially folic acid deficiency. Supplementation has no apparent effect after the sixth week of pregnancy.
4. **Maternal Smoking.** An increase in abruption and fetal deaths occurs in those who smoke more than 10 cigarettes per day.
5. **Cocaine Use**
6. Acute external trauma (rare)
7. Decompression of polyhydramnios (rare)

D. **Recurrence Rate.** A 5%–17% recurrence rate is noted after the first episode of abruption and a 25% rate is seen after the second. Subsequent episodes are usually more severe than the first.

E. Pathophysiology. Maternal hemorrhage occurs in the decidua basalis. In most cases the source of the bleeding is small arterial vessels in the basal layer of the decidua that are pathologically prone to rupture. Infusion of thrombin-rich decidual tissue into the maternal circulation may result in disseminated intravascular coagulation (DIC) (Figs 17–1 to 17–5 and Table 17–2).

F. Perinatal Morbidity and Mortality

1. The perinatal mortality rate is 151/1,000.

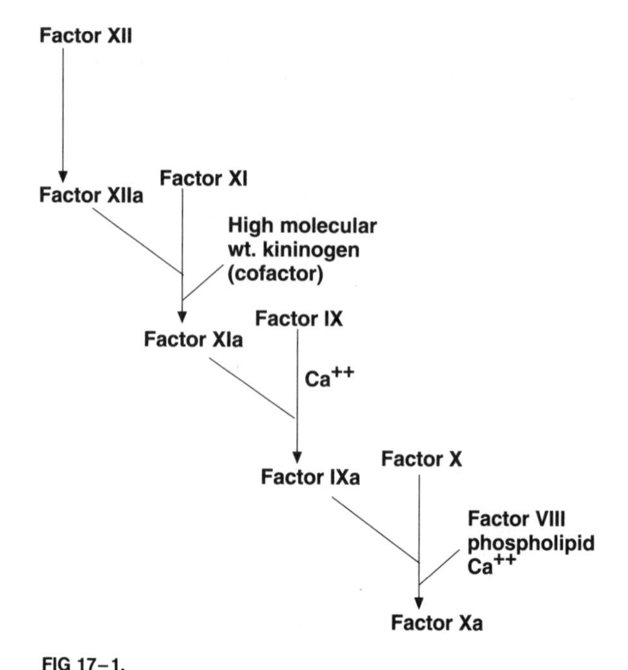

FIG 17–1.

The intrinsic coagulation cascade. (From Beck WS (ed): *Hematology,* ed 3. Cambridge, Mass, The MIT Press, 1981. Used by permission.)

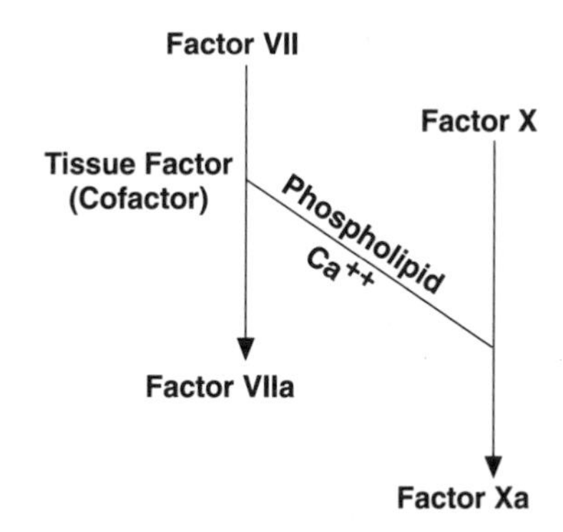

FIG 17–2.
The extrinsic coagulation cascade. (From Beck WS (ed): *Hematology*, ed 3. Cambridge, Mass, The MIT Press, 1981. Used by permission.)

2. Up to 40% of all fetal demises resulting from abruptio placentae occur in gestations with fetuses alive at admission.
3. Neonatal deaths are associated with preterm birth, fetal asphyxia, and fetal exsanguination (rare).
4. Infants are often small for gestational age.
5. Congenital malformations (nonspecific) are increased two to five times more than in the general population for reasons unknown.

G. Maternal Morbidity and Mortality

1. The most common complications are anemia, hemorrhage, shock, DIC, and Couvelaire uterus. As a result of hemorrhagic shock and hypotension, irreversible renal damage may occur. Although rare, uterine rupture may occur. The maternal mortality rate is not increased above that noted in the general pregnant population.
2. Spontaneous abortion occurs in 14% of future pregnancies.
3. Repeated abruption occurs in 9.3% of future pregnancies.
4. Rh sensitization may occur in Rh-negative mothers. Thirty-five percent of patients with blood loss severe enough to require transfusion have evidence of fetal-maternal bleeding. Thus all Rh-negative patients should have

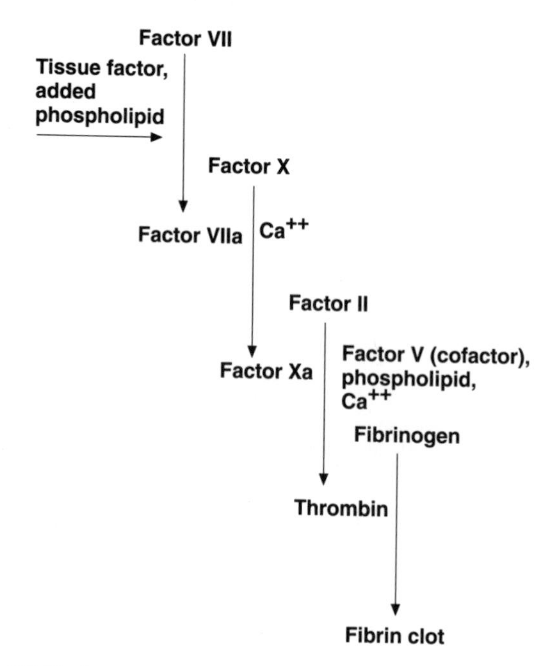

FIG 17–3.
Factors influencing the prothrombin time. (From Beck WS (ed): *Hematology*, ed 3. Cambridge, Mass, The MIT Press, 1981. Used by permission.)

a Kleihauer-Betke performed and, if positive, be given an ampule (300 μg) of RhoGAM.

H. Evaluation

1. **History.** Painful vaginal bleeding, usually associated with uterine contractions
2. **Physical Examination**
   a. The majority of patients present with external bleeding which is characteristically dark and nonclotting (occasionally serosanguineous).
   b. Hypertonic frequent uterine contractions.

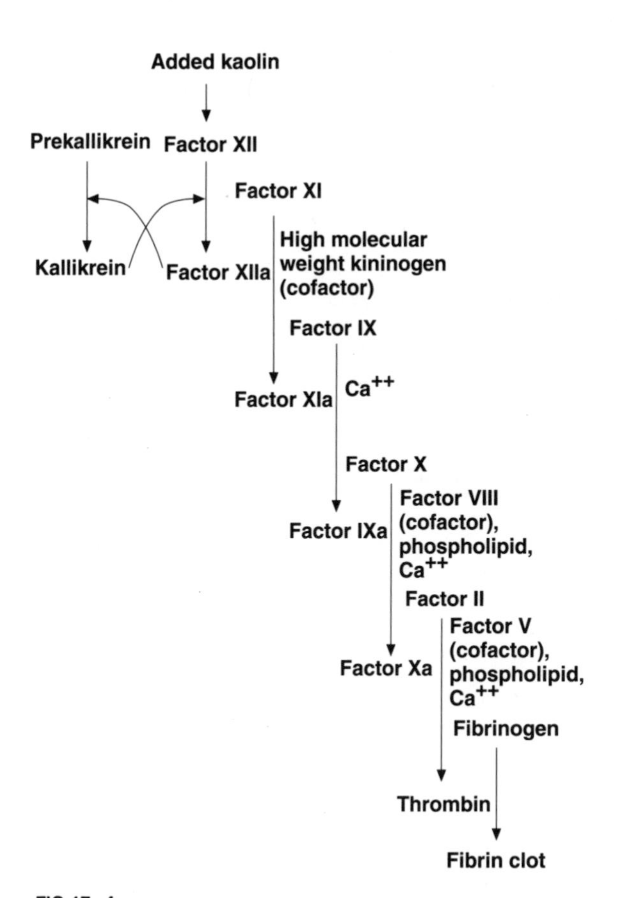

FIG 17–4.
Factors influencing the partial thromboplastin time. (From Beck WS (ed): *Hematology*, ed 3. Cambridge, Mass, The MIT Press, 1981. Used by permission.

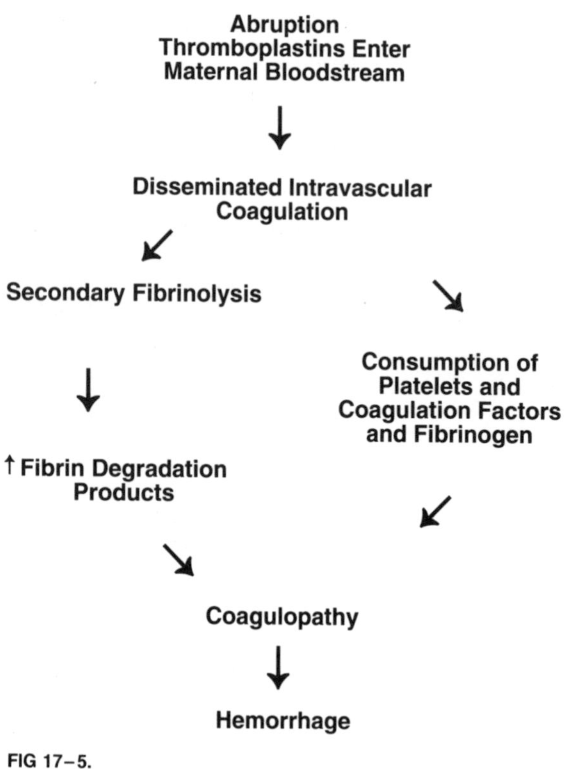

FIG 17–5.
Pathogenesis of the coagulation disorder in abruptio placentae.

   c. Fetal distress.
   d. Tender uterus.
   e. Consider the diagnosis of uterine rupture if shock, diffuse abdominal pain, and tenderness are present (immediate laparotomy is indicated).
3. **Diagnostic Data**
   a. **Ultrasound** is useful to rule out placenta previa. Evidence of a retroplacental blood clot would make the di-

TABLE 17–2.
Conditions Associated With DIC*

Obstetric	Either	Non-obstetric
Abruptio placentae Amniotic fluid embolism Eclampsia and severe preeclampsia Abortion with hyperosmolar urea or saline Retained dead fetus or missed abortion Hydatidiform mole Retained placenta (esp. accreta) Rupture of the uterus Significant fetomaternal hemorrhage	Prolonged shock of any cause Transfusion of incompatible blood Infection (esp. with sepsis): Bacterial, viral, fungal, rickettsial, or protozoal (Most common in obstetrics: Septic abortion or severe chorioamnionitis/endometritis)	Malignancy Extensive surgery Collagen vascular disease CNS trauma Allergic reactions Burns Vascular malformations Pancreatitis Purpura fulminans

*From Main DM, Main EK: *Obstetrics and Gynecology: A Pocket Reference.* St Louis, Mosby–Year Book, 1984. Used by permission.

agnosis, especially in the minority of patients who have a concealed hemorrhage. Presence of a clot on ultrasound may not change management if the patient's condition is stable otherwise. Absence of a clot does not rule out abruption. An ultrasound may also be used to confirm fetal death.

b. **CBC with platelets, fibrinogen,** and, if the possibility of DIC is present, consider prothrombin time, partial thromboplastin time, and fibrinogen degradation products tests. These six laboratory evaluations are often collectively called a **DIC panel.** A fibrinogen level is a good screening test because other tests will not change until after the fibrinogen level falls (Table 17–3).
c. An Apt test (Table 17–4) performed on the blood collected vaginally is often positive for fetal blood, and a Kleihauer-Betke test of maternal venous blood (Table 17–5) also often reveals the presence of fetal blood cells.
d. The minority of patients who have a concealed hemorrhage often present with uterine contractions nonresponsive to tocolysis.

TABLE 17–3.
Coagulation Studies in Abruptio Placentae

Test	Parameter Studied	Normal Value	Value in Abruption
Platelet count	Platelet number	$\geq$150,000/mm^3	Usually decreased
Fibrinogen	Fibrinogen level	400–650 mg/dL	Usually decreased
Fibrin degradation products	Fibrin and fibrinogen degradation products	$<$10 μg/mL	Usually increased
Prothrombin time	Factors II, V, VII, X (the extrinsic and common pathways)	10–12 sec	Normal to prolonged
Partial thromboplastin time	Factors II, V, XIII, IX, X, XI (the intrinsic and common pathways)	24–38 sec	Normal to prolonged
Thrombin time	Factors I, II circulating split-product heparin effect	16–20 sec	Decreased, reflects fibrinogen change
Bleeding time	Vascular integrity and platelet function	1–5 min	Normal—no clinical value in abruption
Whole blood clotting time	Intrinsic and common pathways Platelet function Fibrinolytic activity	Clot formation 4–6 min Retraction: $<$1 hr Lysis: none in 24 hr	Abnormal clot formation indicates severe deficiency Abnormal retraction with thrombocytopenia
RBC morphology	Microangiopathic hemolysis	Absence of RBC distortion or fragmentation	Presence of distortion or fragmentation is uncommon, but identifies a risk for renal cortical necrosis

TABLE 17–4.

APT Test for Fetal Blood*,†

1. Mix 1 part bloody vaginal fluid with 5–10 parts tap water. Centrifuge ×2 minutes. Supernatant must be pink to proceed.
2. Take 5 parts supernatant and mix with 1 part 1% (0.25N) NaOH. Centrifuge ×2 minutes.
3. Interpretation: A pink color indicates fetal blood. A yellow-brown color indicates maternal blood. Adult oxyhemoglobin is less resistant to alkali than fetal oxyhemoglobin. During this reaction adult oxyhemoglobin is converted to alkaline globin hematin.

Alternative method if a centrifuge is not available:

1. Obtain blood from vaginal aspiration.
2. To 2 mL blood (10 drops) add 2 mL H_2O (10 drops and 0.8 mL NaOH (5 drops).
3. Maternal blood will be brown.
4. Fetal blood remains red/pink.

*Modified from Apt L, Downey WS: "Melena" neonatorum: The swallowed blood syndrome, *J Pediatr* 1955; 47:6.

†Used to indicate if bloody amniotic fluid or vaginal blood is fetal in origin.

TABLE 17–5.

Kleihauer-Betke Test for Fetal Hemoglobin†

Principle of test: When red cells are placed in an acid medium (citrate buffer, pH 3.3), fetal hemoglobin is less soluble than adult hemoglobin. This test is usually performed by skilled laboratory technicians. After acid elution, a peripheral smear is prepared. The erythrocytes containing adult hemoglobin A will be recognizable as intact, hemoglobin-free red cell membranes (ghosts), while fetal erythrocytes will still contain hemoglobin.

In theory, this test can detect fetal-maternal bleeds as small as 0.001 ml. In practice, such a clear separation is not possible, because approximately 0.5% of hemoglobin in adults is Hgb F.

There are commercial kits which are rapid, convenient, and quite reliable modifications of the Kleihauer-Betke test. (Fetal-dex [orthodiagnostics] and BMC Reagent Set [Boehringer Mannheim Corp.]).

For further description of the acid elution methods and method of calculating size of fetal-maternal bleed, see:

1. Queenan JT: *Modern Management of the Rh Problem* ed. 2. Hagerstown, MD, Harper & Row, 1977.
2. Scott JR, Warenski JC: Tests to detect and quantitate fetomaternal bleeding, *Clin Obstet Gynecol* 1982; 25:277.

*From Main DM, Main EK: *Obstetrics and Gynecology: A Pocket Reference.* St. Louis, Mosby–Year Book, 1984, p 104. Used by permission.

†Used to screen maternal blood for fetal erythrocytes and hence a significant fetal-maternal bleed.

e. A definitive diagnosis is made upon delivery when gross inspection of the placenta reveals an organized or adherent clot lying within a cup-shaped depression on the maternal surface. This may not be noted if the abruption occurred recently.

4. The classification of abruptio placentae by severity is shown in Table 17–6.
5. The differential diagnosis includes **chorioamnionitis, appendicitis and pyelonephritis.**

I. **Therapeutic Management** (Fig 17–6)

1. **Management of a Patient With Severe Abruptio Placentae and a Fetal Demise:**
   a. Initiate a **blood transfusion,** preferably with fresh whole blood (alternative: packed red blood cells [PRBCs]), (Tables 17–7 and 17–8).
   b. Infuse adequate blood and crystalloid to **maintain Hct >30% and U/O >30 mL/hr.**
   c. Send a **DIC panel:** The patient may have a consumptive coagulopathy.
      1) **Reevaluate for DIC after every 4 units of blood.**

TABLE 17–6.
Classification of Abruptio Placentae by Severity*

	Classification		
Clinical Signs	Mild	Moderate	Severe
Vaginal bleeding	Mild	Mild–moderate	Moderate–severe
Uterine tenderness	None	Slight	Marked
Uterine contractions	Irritable	Irritable vs tetanic	Tetanic and painful
Vital signs	Stable	Tachycardia ± orthostatic BP changes	Unstable
Fetal heart rate	Normal	± Distress	Distress/death
Coagulation studies	Normal	Fibrinogen 150–250 mg/dL	Fibrinogen <150 mg/dL, platelets low, ± disseminated intravascular coagulation

*The clinical picture is often confusing, with some aspects consistent with one grade of abruption and other findings with a different grade.

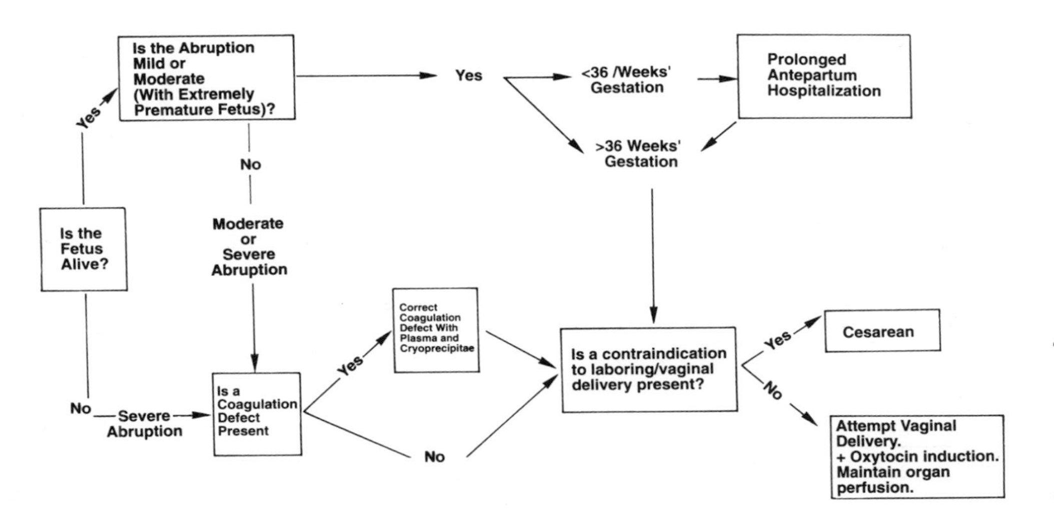

FIG 17–6.
Management of abruptio placentae.

TABLE 17–7.

Comparison of Blood Replacement Products*

Product	Hospital Cost/Unit	Contents	Volume	Effect
Whole blood (WB)	$95	RBC (2.3-DPG) WBC (not functional after 24 hr) Coagulation factors (50%—V, VIII after 7 days) Plasma proteins	500 cc	Increase volume (ml/ml) Increase Hct 3%/unit
Packed red cells	$83	RBC—same as WB WBC—less than WB Plasma proteins—few	240 mL	Same RBC as whole blood Less risk febrile, or WBC transfusion reaction Increase Hct 3%/unit
Platelets	$46	55×10^6 platelets/unit few WBC plasma	50 mL	Increase platelet count 5,000–10,000 μl/unit Give 6 packs minimum
Fresh frozen plasma	$47	Clotting factors V, VIII fibrinogen	250 cc	Only source of factors V, XI, XII Increase fibrinogen 10 mg%/unit
Cryoprecipitate	$35	Factor VIII 25% fibrinogen von Willebrand's factor	40 mL	Increase fibrinogen 10 mg%/unit
Albumin 5%	$312	Albumin	500 mL	
Albumin 25%	$193	Albumin	50 mL	

*From Gabbe SG, Niebyl JR, Simpson JL. *Obstetrics: Normal and Problem Pregnancies.* New York, Churchill Livingstone, 1986. Used by permission.

TABLE 17–8.
Risk of Hepatitis and Acquired Immunodeficiency Syndrome

I. Blood products and the risk of hepatitis and human immunodeficiency virus (HIV)
- **A.** Each blood product unit (whole blood, packed red blood cells, platelets, fresh frozen plasma, platelets, and cryoprecipitate) is from an individual donor.
- **B.** Each unit of a blood product carries the following risks:
  1. Hepatitis C 3%–5%
  2. HIV 1/50,000–1/100,000
- **C.** Albumin is pooled from many donors; thus the risk of the above infections is multiplied many times for each unit administered.

II. Platelets
- **A.** Many hospitals are now offering plateletpheresis. This process allows a patient to receive 8–10 units of platelets from one donor, thus significantly decreasing the hepatitis and HIV infection risks in patients who require large infusions. The cost for 8–10 units of platelets obtained by plateletpheresis is $500.
- **B.** Each unit of platelets will raise the platelet count by about 10,000 in a normal individual. In the idiopathic thrombocytopenic purpura patient, the rise may be much less due to immune destruction of the transfused platelets.

2) Thirty-eight percent of patients with abruptio placentae severe enough to kill a fetus have a plasma **fibrinogen** level <150 mg/dL, and 28% have a level <100 mg/dL.
3) Screening for a clinically significant coagulopathy:
   a) Observe a 5 mL clot tube. If the blood fails to clot within 6 minutes, or if the clot fails to retract and lyse within 2 hours, a marked coagulopathy is present.
   Action in terms of ordering appropriate replacement products need not await confirmatory tests.
   b) Strongly consider using fresh frozen plasma or cryoprecipitate (they take 60 minutes to prepare) to replace fibrinogen and clotting factors, especially if a cesarean section or an episiotomy is performed. Transfuse adequate fresh frozen plasma or cryoprecipitate to

achieve a fibrinogen level of 100–150 mg/dL. If platelets are needed, transfuse to a count of >100,000/μL.

c) A vaginal delivery may be performed in the presence of very low clotting factors if unusual trauma is avoided.

4) Attempt a vaginal delivery of the fetus regardless of fetal presentation if the patient is in stable condition and no other obstetric indications for a cesarean are present.
5) **Oxytocin Induction.** If adequate spontaneous labor is not present, consider using oxytocin for induction or augmentation of labor according to your hospital's protocol.
6) If the maternal status is deteriorating despite blood product replacement, proceed to a cesarean delivery (the mother must be hemodynamically stable before surgery is performed). This should rarely be necessary.
7) After delivery of the fetus and placenta, the coagulopathy will resolve within hours with appropriate blood replacement and maintenance of intravascular pressure.
8) Place a Foley catheter to gravity.
9) Start oxygen at 8 L/min via a nasal cannula.
10) If the U/O is <30 mL/hr, or if the patient's hemodynamic status is unstable, consider placing a peripheral capillary venous pressure (CVP) line or central monitoring with a Swan-Ganz catheter. Normal values are CVP = 5–10 cm H_2O; pulmonary capillary wedge pressure = 3–10 mm Hg.
11) In cases of shock, place an arterial line to monitor the patient's **BP.**

2. **Management of the Patient With a Live Fetus**

a. **Severe Abruption**

1) Type and cross 4 units of packed red blood cells.
2) Prepare for a cesarean unless special circumstances are present (maternal shock, previable fetus). A cesarean should be performed only after the patient is in stable condition, with blood products infusing, even in the face of fetal distress.
3) A severe abruption results in increased maternal mortality and morbidity.

b. **Moderate Abruption**
   1) Perform an amniotomy and initiate an oxytocin induction if indicated (if no reason for a cesarean exists).
   2) The patient with a moderate abruption has an excellent prospect for a vaginal delivery with good fetal and maternal outcomes.
   3) If the uterus becomes hypertonic during labor, or if signs of fetal distress appear, assume extension of the abruption and deliver immediately, by cesarean if necessary.
   4) If the baby is extremely premature, selective patients may be considered for transfusion and delayed delivery versus expectant management.

c. **Mild Abruption With an Immature Fetus**
   1) Observe on labor and delivery.
   2) When the conditions of the patient and the fetus are assessed to be stable, transfer the patient to the antepartum floor for long-term antepartum care (see IVC4).

IV. Placenta Previa

A. Background

1. **Definition**

   a. Placenta previa is classified according to the degree to which the os is covered by the placenta. This classification is based on ultrasound findings or a double setup examination:
      1) **Total:** The internal os is completely covered by placental tissue.
      2) **Partial:** The internal os is partially covered by placental tissue.
      3) **Marginal:** The edge of the placenta is at the margin of the internal os but covers no portion of the os.
      4) **Lateral or Low Lying:** The edge of the placenta may be palpated by a finger introduced through the cervix.

   b. The amount of **blood loss** directly correlates with the degree of previa, but not with the number of bleeding episodes or perinatal mortality. The origin of blood loss is presumed to be maternal.

2. **Etiology**
   a. No specific cause has been identified.
   b. Conditions associated with an increased prevalence of placenta previa include:
      1) Increased parity (It is thought that previous gestations permanently damage the endometrium, making every area of placental attachment unsuitable for placental attachment in subsequent pregnancies.)
      2) Closely spaced pregnancies
      3) Previous abortion
      4) Previous cesarean section
      5) Multiple gestations
      6) Advanced maternal age
      7) Anemia
      8) Abnormal fetal presentation
      9) Congenital malformations
      10) Tumors that distort contour of uterus
      11) Endometritis
      12) Male fetus
3. **Incidence**
   a. The incidence is:
      1) 1/250 pregnancies beyond 24 weeks
      2) 1/1,500 nulliparas
      3) 1/20 grand multiparas
   b. The frequency of the different classes of placenta previa includes:
      1) Total previa 23%–31%
      2) Partial previa 21%–33%
      3) Marginal previa 37%–55%
   c. The incidence is affected by the **gestational age** at the time of diagnosis.
      1) The ultrasound diagnosis of placenta previa in the second trimester is 5% to 15%.
      2) The ultrasound diagnosis of placenta previa at term is 0.5%. (The 90% conversion rate is thought to result from differential growth of the uterus.)
      3) If an ultrasound at 26–28 weeks demonstrates a placenta previa, it will most likely persist until the delivery, and thus the patient should be managed expectantly (pelvic rest, no heavy work).

d. The **recurrence rate** for placenta previa is 12 times the expected incidence.

4. **Perinatal Morbidity and Mortality**
   a. The perinatal mortality rate is less than 10% to 15%.
   b. Prematurity is the primary cause of perinatal morbidity and mortality. An increased perinatal mortality rate is associated with early bleeding, larger blood losses, and larger placenta previas (i.e., complete versus marginal).
   c. **Congenital malformations** (nonspecific) are two to four times more frequent in patients with placenta previa.
5. **Maternal Morbidity and Mortality**
   a. The maternal mortality rate is less than 1%.
   b. Placenta accreta occurs in 4% of patients with placenta previa, and in 25% of those with placenta previa and a prior cesarean. Treatment is hysterectomy unless the attachment is limited and the bleeding controlled with local sutures.
   c. Abruptio placentae recurs more frequently than in the general population (5% to 17% recurrence rate).
   d. Rh sensitization may occur in Rh-negative mothers. Thirty-five percent of patients with blood loss severe enough to require transfusion have evidence of a fetal-maternal bleeding. Thus all Rh-negative patients should have a Kleihauer-Betke performed and, if positive, should be given an ampule (300 μg) of RhoGAM.
   e. DIC rarely occurs, and when it does it usually results from hemorrhagic shock or abruptio placentae.
   f. Irreversible renal damage is rare, but is the most common long-term complication of hemorrhagic shock and hypotension.

B. Evaluation

1. **Clinical Presentation**
   a. **Vaginal bleeding,** usually painless, of sudden onset in the second or third trimester
      1) The peak incidence is at 34 weeks' gestation; 65% of patients have their first bleeding after 30 weeks. No maternal fatality has been associated with the first bleeding episode (barring an inap-

propriate vaginal examination, which may result in a massive maternal hemorrhage).

a) Bleeding may begin without an obvious inciting cause (i.e., vaginal examination, intercourse, onset of labor). In these cases, it may be precipitated by formation of the lower uterine segment with consequent detachment of a portion of the placenta.

b) In 10% of cases bleeding begins only with the onset of labor.

b. **Abnormal Fetal Presentation.** Abnormal fetal presentations are increased in the presence of placenta previa at the following rates.

1) Breech, shoulder, and compound presentations occur in up to 35% of placenta previa cases.

2) 60% of all transverse lies are associated with placenta previa.

3) 24% of all breech and compound lies are associated with placenta previa.

2. **Diagnostic Evaluation**

a. **Ultrasound** provides a 98% accuracy rate in localizing the placenta. In a small percentage of patients ultrasound cannot unequivocally diagnose placenta previa. (In these patients a double setup examination may be indicated.) This usually occurs beyond 32 weeks when elevation of the presenting part is essential for obtaining adequate resolution.

1) Areas of ultrasound confusion include a blood clot at the level of the internal os, the presence of a succenturiate lobe, or a thick "decidual reaction."

2) The diagnosis is confirmed by finding the placenta covering at least a portion of the cervix at the time of a double setup examination or cesarean section.

b. A **gentle speculum examination** should be performed for evaluation of the vagina and cervix upon admission, and intermittently as indicated.

C. **Management of Placenta Previa**

1. **Severe Hemorrhage**

a. Place **two large-bore IVs,** one for Ringer's lactate, the second for blood.

b. Blood samples to be drawn upon admission:
   1) DIC panel (CBC, prothrombin time, partial thromboplastin time, platelets, fibrinogen, and fibrinogen degradation products).
   2) Type and crossmatch for four units of PRBCs.
   3) If necessary, start infusing **O-negative blood** immediately. Keep the Blood Bank informed of the patient's status. Infuse **type-specific** blood as soon as it is available.
   4) Type-specific blood takes 15 to 30 minutes to prepare.
   5) A complete crossmatch requires 45 to 60 minutes to prepare if no major antibodies are found.
   6) Keep **4 units of PRBCs** available at all times.
   7) Fresh whole blood, platelets, and cryoprecipitate (rarely) may be necessary.

c. Place a Foley catheter and treat a decreased U/O aggressively, maintaining U/O ≥30 mL/hr. Hydrate the patient adequately. Later, if indicated, give a 20–60 mg bolus of furosemide (Lasix). Hypovolemic shock may result in acute tubular and cortical necrosis.

d. Consider placing a peripheral **CVP** or a central **Swan-Ganz** catheter for accurate assessment of fluid status.

e. Perform an ultrasound for gestational dating.

f. Deliver by cesarean.

2. **Moderate Hemorrhage.** When the acute bleeding episode has subsided and the maternal condition has stabilized, evaluate fetal lung maturity for all gestations between 32 and 36 weeks. Assume pulmonary immaturity if the gestation is <32 weeks, maturity if >36 weeks.

   a. **Mature.** Deliver immediately.

   b. **Immature**
      1) Provide intensive care on labor and delivery for the first 24–48 hours. Maintain Hb ≥10 g/dL (Hct ≥30). Consider using steroids to accelerate fetal lung maturation.
      2) Tocolyse with $MgSO_4$ if the uterus is irritable or if preterm labor develops.
      3) If the patient's condition remains unstable with steady moderate blood loss, or if the patient requires more than 2 units of blood in 24 hours, deliver.

4) If the patient's condition becomes stable and remains so for 24–48 hours, she is a candidate for long-term antepartum care. Most patients will fit into this category.

3. **Mild Bleeding**
   a. If the fetus is mature (>36 weeks), deliver.
   b. In the patient whose fetus is <36 weeks' gestation with a mature lung profile, whose bleeding ceases, and who has no need for transfusion, consider delaying delivery.
   c. If the fetal lungs are immature, the patient may receive long-term antepartum care.
4. **Long-term Antepartum Care**
   a. **Patient Selection.** Patients with proved fetal pulmonary immaturity, and those with gestations ≤36 weeks, stable vital signs, and resolution of bleeding, are eligible.
   b. **Continuous hospitalization** for a minimum of 72 hours is advised because nearly one third of all patients with placenta previa who are initially selected for expectant management will require delivery within this time.
   c. **Orders for the Floor**
      1) Bed rest with bathroom privileges
      2) Stool softeners
      3) Prenatal vitamins, $FeSO_4$
      4) Laboratory tests:
         a) Obtain Hb weekly; keep Hb ≥10 g/dL).
         b) For patients with placenta previa, type and hold 2 units PRBCs. Have this available at all times. Blood specimens for type and hold will probably need to be drawn every 2–3 days.
      5) Antepartum testing if indicated
      6) Daily uterine monitoring if indicated
   d. Perform an amniocentesis for fetal pulmonary studies at 36 weeks and if fetal lungs are immature, repeat every 7 to 10 days. When fetal lungs are mature, the patient with placenta previa should be scheduled for a cesarean delivery.
   e. If the patient has had no further bleeding and this was her first admission for bleeding, she may go home at strict bed and pelvic rest after being observed for 72 hours on the antepartum floor, if:

1) She lives within 15 minutes of the hospital.
2) Has a responsible adult who will be at home with her.
3) The companion has access to an automobile 24 hours a day.

V. Vasa Previa

A. Definition. Umbilical vessels insert velamentously in a low-lying placenta and traverse the membranes in front of the fetal presenting part.

B. Pathology. The vessels are not protected by Wharton's jelly.

C. Incidence

1. Vasa previa occurs in 0.1%–1.8% of all pregnancies, with the trend toward the lower end of this range.
2. Singletons: 0.25%–1.25%.
3. Twins: 6%–10%.
4. Triplets: 95%.

D. Perinatal mortality is greater than 50%, resulting from a vasa previa tear or rupture with resultant fetal exsanguination. Compression of the fetal vessels by the presenting part may cause hypoxia and eventual death.

E. Diagnosis

1. Painless vaginal bleeding is common, but not mandatory for the diagnosis.

TABLE 17–9.
Relationship of Signs and Treatment Modalities to Differential Diagnosis

Signs and Treatment Modalities	Differential Diagnosis		
	Previa	Abruption	Vasa Previa
Pain with uterine contractions	No	Yes	No
Tender uterus	No	Yes	No
Primary danger	Mother	Fetus/mother	Fetus
Blood	Maternal	Maternal	Fetal
Ultrasound helpful	Yes	Maybe	Yes
Cesarean mandatory	Yes	No	Yes

2. **Fetal Bleeding—Diagnosis**
   a. Examination of blood for nucleated RBCs, normoblasts
   b. Hemoglobin electrophoresis (takes 60 minutes)
   c. Apt test (see Table 17–4)
3. Fetal distress is a common presentation. Frequently seen fetal heart rate patterns include sinusoidal changes, tachycardia, late decelerations, or prolonged decelerations.

F. Treatment is an emergent cesarean section.

VI. Summary. Relationship of signs and treatment modalities to differential diagnosis is shown in Table 17–9.

BIBLIOGRAPHY

Arias F: *High Risk Pregnancy and Delivery*. St Louis, Mosby–Year Book, 1984.

Bond AL, Edersheim TG, Curry L, et al: Expectant management of abruptio placentae before 35 weeks' gestation. *Am J Perinatol* 1989; 6(2):121.

Cotton DB, Read JA, Paul RH, et al: The conservative aggressive management of placenta previa. *Am J Obstet Gynecol* 1980; 137(6):687.

Cunningham FG, MacDonald PC, Gant NF: *William's Obstetrics*, ed 17. Norwalk, Conn, Appleton-Century-Crofts, 1985.

Hibbard BM, Jeffcoate TNA: Abruptio placentae. *Obstet Gynecol* 1966; 27(2):155.

Higgins SD, Garite TJ: Late abruptio placenta in trauma patients. Implications for Monitoring. *Obstet Gynecol* 1984; 63(3)suppl:105.

Karegard M, Gennser G: Incidence and recurrence rate of abruptio placentae in Sweden. *Obstet Gynecol* 1986; 67(4):523.

McShane PM, Heyl PS, Epstein MF: Maternal and perinatal morbidity resulting from placenta previa. *Obstet Gynecol* 1985; 65(2):176.

Sampson MB, Lastres O, Tomasi AM, et al: Tocolysis with terbutaline sulfate in patients with placenta previa complicated by premature labor. *J Repro Med* 1984; 29(4):248.

Sholl JS: Abruptio placentae: Clinical management in nonacute cases, *Am J Obstet Gynecol* 156(1):40–51; 1987.

MULTIPLE GESTATION

18

I. Background

A. Definitions

1. **Monozygotic** (MZ) twins occur in the event of the cleavage of one fertilized egg.
2. **Dizygotic** (DZ) twins result from the fertilization of two ova.
3. **Placental morphology** (described in terms of membranes) (Fig 18–1)
   a. Dichorionic diamniotic (fused)
   b. Dichorionic diamniotic (separated)
   c. Monochorionic monoamniotic
   d. Monochorionic diamniotic

B. Incidence

1. Of all US births, 1.5% are multiple gestations. The ratio of multiple gestations to singleton births are:
   a. Twins 1:90
   b. Triplets 1:8,000
   c. Quadruplets 1:700,000
2. MZ twins occur in 4/1,000 births and account for one third of all multiple gestations. The occurrence rate of MZ twinning is independent of race, maternal age, and parity.
3. DZ twinning is more frequent in certain families. It is most common in blacks, least common in Asians, and the rate of DZ twinning increases with maternal age, parity, height, weight, and the use of fertility drugs.

C. Perinatal Morbidity and Mortality

1. Perinatal mortality in multiple gestations is 2 to 5 times that of singleton pregnancies.
2. The mortality rate of MZ twins is 2 to 3 times greater than that of DZ twins.
3. Prematurity accounts for the greater portion of mortality and morbidity. Other factors that play a significant role

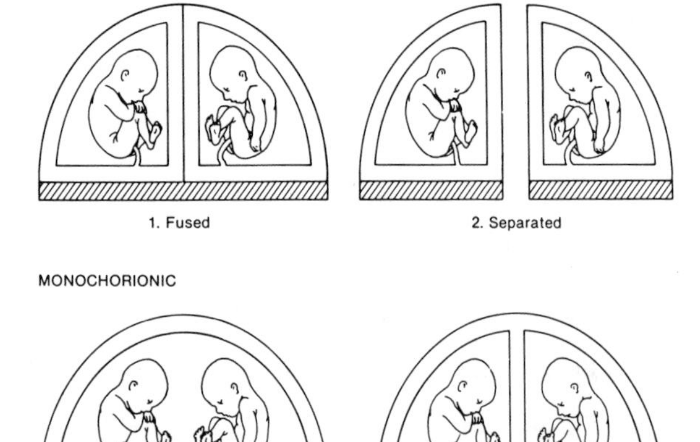

FIG 18–1.
Placental morphology in twin pregnancy. (From Arias F: *High-Risk Pregnancy and Delivery*. St Louis, Mosby–Year Book, 1984. Used by permission.)

are intrauterine growth retardation, (IUGR), stillbirth, congenital anomalies, hydramnios, vasa previa, pregnancy-induced hypertension (PIH), and placenta previa.

a. Discordant IUGR may result from twin-twin transfusion or placental steal.
b. Stillbirth may result from cord accidents or factors relating to IUGR if present.
c. Congenital anomalies occur at twice the rate (per twin) of singletons.
d. Hydramnios and vasa previa are more frequent in multiple gestations.
e. PIH and placenta previa may complicate the maternal status. These are seen with increased frequency in multiple gestations and may result in a premature delivery.

f. Individual twins and singletons have similar weights up to 32 weeks' gestation, after which the twins weigh less individually than the singleton.

g. **Discordant Growth.** No standard definition can be found for this term. This is a pediatric diagnosis referring to the difference in birth weights as a percentage of the larger twin's weight. The definition ranges from 15%–25%, with an incidence of 4%–23%. All studies agree that larger discordances result in higher perinatal mortality. In obstetrics we may attempt to identify this problem early so that we may either reverse it or at least minimize its effects. Ultrasonically, abdominal circumferences or estimated fetal weights (EFWs) by various published formulas are the most reliable comparisons. Differences ≥20% are considered significant, and, when present, **antepartum testing** should be initiated. Ultrasound evaluations should be performed at 26 weeks and every 3–4 weeks thereafter to rule out discordance in all twins.

D. **Maternal Morbidity and Mortality.** The maternal mortality rate is not increased above that noted in the general population; however, women with multiple pregnancies are at a greater risk for PIH, placenta previa, abruptio placentae, hydramnios, and postpartum hemorrhage. Most importantly, there is an increased risk of preterm labor.

II. Evaluation

A. **Diagnosis.** It is estimated that among 20%–40% of twins with prenatal care diagnosis of multiple gestation was not made until delivery. Current ultrasound techniques, however, should have a diagnosis rate of about 90% with physician awareness. An ultrasound evaluation for determination of a multiple gestation should be undertaken if any of the following are found:

1. Uterine fundal height is more than 3 cm greater than the gestational age in weeks.
2. There is a family history of twins.
3. The patient has a history of taking ovulation-inducing agents (i.e., clomiphene, pituitary gonadotropins).

B. **Pulmonary Maturity.** Concordant twins have similar pulmonary maturity studies. In discordant twins, the smaller twin is postulated to be more stressed, resulting in a more mature lung; therefore the larger twin will probably have the less mature lung profile (lecithin/sphingomyelin ratio).

C. **Presentations**

1. Vertex/vertex 40%
2. Vertex/breech 26%
3. Breech/vertex 10%
4. Breech/breech 10%
5. Vertex/transverse 8%
6. Miscellaneous 6%

III. Therapeutic Management: Delivery of Diamniotic Twins

A. **Determination of Mode of Delivery.** If the estimated fetal weight of each twin is <1,500 g and the presentation of these twins is other than vertex/vertex, or if triplets/quadruplets are present, better outcomes (umbilical venous pH, Apgar scores) are achieved by cesarean delivery.

1. The majority of studies report that in twins of all gestational ages vertex/vertex twins may be delivered safely vaginally.
2. For fetuses weighing >1,500 g, presentations other than vertex/vertex may be indications for cesarean section, although this is not always necessary. Concordant vertex/breech or vertex/transverse presentations may be delivered vaginally, with twin B delivered either by external cephalic version, total breech extraction, or as a frank breech.
3. If a vaginal delivery of a breech twin B is anticipated, the EFW should be at least 2,000 g to accommodate for a 15% error in estimation (assuring that the true fetal weight is ≥1,500 g). Twin B should not be significantly larger than twin A if breech or transverse, and a vaginal delivery is to be tried.
4. An ultrasound machine should be present in the delivery room for all vaginal deliveries to confirm twin B's presentation after delivery of twin A, and to assist with monitoring the fetus during an external cephalic version. The delivery should be performed in the cesarean section room with immediate availability of a surgical team and equipment.

B. **Labor.** Most patients will enter into labor spontaneously. Because of the high incidence of fetal/maternal complications with multiple gestations, it may be necessary to induce labor with oxytocin (Pitocin) after an abnormal fetal position has been ruled out.

C. **Anesthesia.** An epidural or caudal block is the method of choice for the following reasons:
   1. The patient is unlikely to involuntarily push a small first twin through an incompletely dilated cervix if analgesia is present.
   2. If internal manipulation is necessary, adequate regional analgesia facilitates delivery of the second twin without delay.

D. **Requirements for Attempted Vaginal Delivery**
   1. Recent ultrasound determination of fetal measurements, EFWs, and positions
   2. Crossmatched blood
   3. Dual fetal monitoring throughout labor and delivery
   4. Ultrasound machine in the delivery room
   5. A second obstetrician at the delivery
   6. Two pediatric teams and two warmers available in the neonatal intensive care unit
   7. A second set of clamps and bulb syringe
   8. Pitocin infusion ready in delivery room for administration after the birth of first twin, if spontaneous uterine contractions become incoordinate

E. **Delivery of First Twin.** Do not obtain cord blood from the first cord unless it is double clamped.

F. **Delivery of Second Twin**
   1. Potential problems:
      a. Delayed delivery
      b. Prolonged anesthesia
      c. Cord prolapse
      d. Placental separation
      e. Operative delivery
   2. If a vaginal delivery from a vertex presentation is planned, guide the head into the pelvis, rupture the second membrane (if present). Apply a scalp electrode. If a frank breech delivery is planned, glide the buttocks into the pelvis, rupture the second membrane, and apply an electrode to a buttock (for heart rate monitoring). If the fetal heart rate is normal, hemorrhage is not present, and the cord does not present, there is no need to dramatically expedite the delivery. If the patient's own expulsive efforts are inadequate (uterine contractions incoordinate), initiate Pitocin augmentation of labor.

3. If no complications arise, one may wait at least 2–3 hours, with Pitocin augmentation of labor as necessary, for delivery of the second twin before diagnosing cephalopelvic disproportion or failure to progress.

BIBLIOGRAPHY

Arias F: *High-Risk Pregnancy and Delivery*. St Louis, Mosby–Year Book, 1984, p 264.

Blickstein I, Schwartz-Shoham F, Cancet M, et al: Vaginal delivery of the second twin in breech presentation. *Obstet Gynecol* 1987; 69:774.

Cetrulo CL: The controversy of mode of delivery of twins: The intrapartum management of twin gestation (Part I). *Semin Perinatol* 1986; 10:39.

Chervenak FA: The controversy of mode of delivery of twins: The intrapartum management of twin gestation (Part II). *Semin Perinatol* 1986; 10:44.

Creasy RK, Resnik R: *Maternal-Fetal Medicine,* Philadelphia, WB Saunders, 1984.

Gocke SE, Nageotte MP, Garite TJ, et al: Management of the nonvertex second twin: Primary cesarean section, external version, or primary breech extraction. *Am J Obstet Gynecol* 1989; 161:111–114.

Mishell DR, Brenner PF: *Management of Common Problems in Obstetrics and Gynecology*. Oradell, NJ, Medical Economics, 1989.

Rabinovic J, Bankai G, Reichman B, et al: Randomized management of the second non-vertex twin: Vaginal delivery or cesarean section. *Am J Obstet Gynecol* 1987; 156:52.

PART IV

APPENDICES

MATERNAL PHYSIOLOGY

APPENDIX A: TEMPERATURE CONVERSION CHART*

TABLE A–1.

To Convert Centigrade to Fahrenheit: (9/5 × Temperature) + 32
To Convert Fahrenheit to Centigrade: (Temperature − 32) × 5/9
Temperature Equivalents

Centigrade	Fahrenheit	Centigrade	Fahrenheit
35.0	95.0	38.2	100.7
35.2	95.4	38.4	101.1
35.4	95.7	38.6	101.4
35.6	96.1	38.8	101.8
35.8	96.4	39.0	102.2
36.0	96.8	39.2	102.5
36.2	97.1	39.4	102.9
36.4	97.5	39.6	103.2
36.6	97.8	39.8	103.6
36.8	98.2	40.0	104.0
37.0	98.6	40.2	104.3
37.2	98.9	40.4	104.7
37.4	99.3	40.6	105.1
37.6	99.6	40.8	105.4
37.8	100.0	41.0	105.8
38.0	100.4	41.2	106.1

*From Main DM, Main EK: *Obstetrics and Gynecology. A Pocket Reference.* St Louis, Mosby–Year Book, 1984. Used by permission.

APPENDIX B: COMMON LABORATORY VALUES IN PREGNANCY*

TABLE B–1.

Test	Normal Range (Non-pregnant)*	Change in Pregnancy†	Timing
Serum chemistries			
Albumin	3.5–4.8 gm/100 mL	↓ 1.0 gm/100 mL	Most by 20 wk, then gradual
Bilirubin			
Total	0.25–1.5 mg/100 mL	No sig. change	
Direct	0–0.2 mg/100 mL	No sig. change	
Blood gases (arterial, whole blood)			
pH	7.35–7.45	No sig. change	
PO_2	80–105 mm Hg	↑ 7 mm Hg	By end of first trimester
PCO_2	35–45 mm Hg	↓ 7 mm Hg	By end of first trimester
Calcium			
Total	9.0–10.3 mg/100 mL	↓ 10%	Gradual fall
Free	4.5–5.0 mg/100 mL	↓ slight	
Carbon dioxide content	24–32 mEq/L	↓ 4–5 mEq/L	By 12 wk, then stable
Ceruloplasmin	15–16 mg/100 mL	↑ 75%	Gradual rise
Chloride	95–105 mEq/L	No sig. change	
Copper	70–155 gm/100 mL	↑ 75%	Gradual rise
Complement (total)	150–250 CH50	↑ 25%	Gradual rise
C3	690–1,470 mg/L	↑ 40%–50%	Gradual rise
C4	105–305 mg/L	No data—probably behaves like C3	

Creatinine (female)	.6–1.1 mg/100 mL	↓ 0.3 mg/100 mL	Most by 20 wk
Fibrinogen	1.5–3.6 gm/L	↑ 1–2 gm/L	Progressive
Folate			
Serum	3 ng/mL	↓ 50%	Gradual fall
Red cell	117–541 ng/mL	↓ 12%	Gradual fall
Glucose, fasting (plasma)	65–105 mg/100 mL	↓ 10%	Gradual fall
Ferritin	15–300 μg/L	↓ 40–50 μg/L	Second trimester, less in supplemented women
Immunoglobulin			
IgA	39–358 mg/100 mL	No sig. change	
IgM	33–229 mg/100 mL	No sig. change	
IgG	679–1,537 mg/100 mL	↓ 100 mg/100 mL	Gradual
Iron (female)	60–135 gm/100 mL	↓ 35%	Gradual, less with supplements
Iron binding capacity	250–350 gm/100 mL	↑ 40%–50%	Second trimester
Lactate (plasma)	0.3–1.3 mmol/L	No change	
Lipids			
Cholesterol	120–330 mg/100 mL	↑ 60–80 mg/100 mL	Progressive after 13 wk
Triglyceride	10–190 mg/100 mL	↑ 100 mg/100 mL	Progressive
Magnesium	1.5–2.4 mEq/L 1.8–2.9 mg/dL	↓ 10%–20%	By 20 wk, then stable
Osmolality	270–290 mOsm/kg	↓ 10 mOsm/kg	By 8 wk, then stable
Phosphorus, inorganic	2.5–6.0 mg/100 mL	No sig. change	
Potassium (plasma)	3.5–4.5 mEq/L	↓ 0.2–0.3 mEq/L	By 20 wk
Protein electrophoresis			
Albumin	3.5–4.8 gm/100 mL	↓ 1.0 gm/100 mL	Most by 20 wk, then gradual
Alpha-1-globulin	0.1–0.5 gm/100 mL	↑ 0.1 gm/100 mL	Gradual
Alpha-2-globulin	0.3–1.2 gm/100 mL	↑ 0.1 gm/100 mL	Gradual

(Continued.)

TABLE B–1 (CONT.).

Test	Normal Range (Non-pregnant)*	Change in Pregnancy†	Timing
Beta globulin	0.7–1.7 gm/100 mL	↑ 0.3 gm/100 mL	Gradual
Gamma globulin	0.7–1.7 gm/100 mL	↓ 0.1 gm/100 mL	Gradual
Protein (total)	6.5–8.5 gm/100 mL	↓ 1.0 gm/100 mL	By 20 wk, then stable
Sodium	135–145 mEq/L	↓ 2–4 mEq/L	By 20 wk, then stable
Urea nitrogen	12–30 mg/100 mL	↓ 50%	First trimester
Uric acid	3.5–8.0 mg/100 mL	↓ 33%	First trimester, rise at term
Urinary chemistries			
Creatinine	15–25 mg/kg/day (1.0–1.4 gm/day)	No sig. change	
Protein	Up to 150 mg/day	Up to 250–300 mg/day	By 20 wk
Creatinine clearance	90–130 ml/min per 1.73 m^2	↑ 40%–50%	By 16 wk
Serum enzymatic activities			
Amylase	23–84 IU/L	↑ 50%–100%	←Controversial
Creatinine phosphokinase	25–145 mU/mL	↓ 25% to 30%	8–20 wk, then returns to normal
Lactic dehydrogenase (LDH)	90–250 mU/mL	Slight ↑, not sig.	
Lipase	4–24 IU/100 mL	↓ 50%	Gradual
Phosphatase, alkaline	30–95 mU/mL	↑ by 100%–200%	Mostly in third trimester
Transaminase			
Alanine amino (SGPT)	5–35 mU/mL	No sig. change	
Aspartate amino (SGOT)	5–40 mU/mL	No sig. change	
Gamma-glutamyl transpeptidase	1–45 IU/L	No sig. change	

Hematologic studies			
Coagulation studies			
Bleeding time (template)	2.5–9.5 min	No sig. change	
Partial thromboplastin time	24–36 sec	No sig. change	
Prothrombin time	70%–100%	No sig. change	
Thrombin time	11.3–18.5 sec	No sig. change	
Factors			
VIII, VIII antigen	60%–160%	↑ 100%–150%	Beginning second trimester
X, IX	60%–160%	↑ 30%	Gradual
VII, XII	60%–160%	No change	Controversial
II, V, XI	60%–160%	No sig. change	
V	60%–160%	↓ 30%	Gradual
Hematocrit (female)	37%–47%	↓ 4%–6%	Bottoms at 30–34 wk
Hemoglobin (female)	12.0–16.0 gm/100 mL	↓ 1.5–2.0 gm/100 mL	Bottoms at 30–34 wk
Erythrocyte count (female)	4.2–10.9 $\times 10^6/mm^3$	↓ 0.8 $\times 10^6/mm^3$	Bottoms at 30–34 wk
Leukocyte count	4.8–10.8 $\times 10^3/mm^3$	↑ 3.5 $\times 10^3/mm^3$	Gradual
polymorphs	48%–82%	↑ 3.0 $\times 10^3/mm^3$	Gradual
lymphocytes	8%–44%	↑ 0.3 $\times 10^3/mm^3$	Gradual
monocytes	2%–8%	No sig. change	
eosinophils	0%–6%	No sig. change	
Platelet count	150–400 $\times 10^3/mm^3$	Slight ↓	
Erythrocyte indexes			
Mean corpuscular hemoglobin (MCH)	27–31 pg/cell	No sig. change	
Mean corpuscular hemoglobin concentration (MCHC)	32–36 gm/dL	No sig. change	
Mean corpuscular volume (MCV)	81–99 cu μ	No sig. change	

(Continued.)

TABLE B–1.

Test	Normal Range (Non-pregnant)*	Change in Pregnancy†	Timing
Sedimentation rate (female)			
Whole blood (Westergren)	Up to 20 mm/hr	↑ 2–6 X	Most by 20 wk, then gradual
Citrated	Up to 10 mm/hr	↑ 3–9 X	Most by 20 wk, then gradual
Serum hormone values			
ACTH	20–100 pg/mL	No sig. change	Early, gradual after 24 wk
Aldosterone	20–90 ng/L	↑ 300%–800%	Gradual
Cortisol (plasma)	8–21 μg/100 mL	↑ 20 μg/100 mL	
Growth hormone, fasting	5 ng/mL	No sig. change	
Insulin, fasting	10 mU/L	No sig. change	First 1/2 of pregnancy
		Slight ↑ (?)	Second 1/2 of pregnancy
Parathyroid hormone	2–10 U/mL	↑ 200%–300%	Progressive after 24 wk
Prolactin (female)	25 ng/mL	↑ 50–400 ng/mL	Gradual, peaks at term
Renin activity (plasma)	0.9–3.3 ng/mL/hr	↑ 100%	Early, stable
Thyroxine, total (T_4)	5.0–11.0 gm/100 mL	↑ 5 mg/100 mL	Early sustained
T_3 resin uptake	35%–45%	↓ to 25%–35%	Early sustained
Free thyroxine index (T_7)	1.75–4.95	No sig. change	
Triiodothyronine (T_3)	125–245 ng/100 mL	↑ 50%	Early sustained
TSH	Up to 8 U/mL	No sig. change	
Free T_4	1–2.3 ng/100 mL	No sig. change	

*From Main DM, Main EK: *Obstetrics and Gynecology. A Pocket Reference.* St Louis, Mosby–Year Book, 1984. Used by permission.

APPENDIX C: ANALGESIA AND ANESTHESIA IN LABOR AND DELIVERY

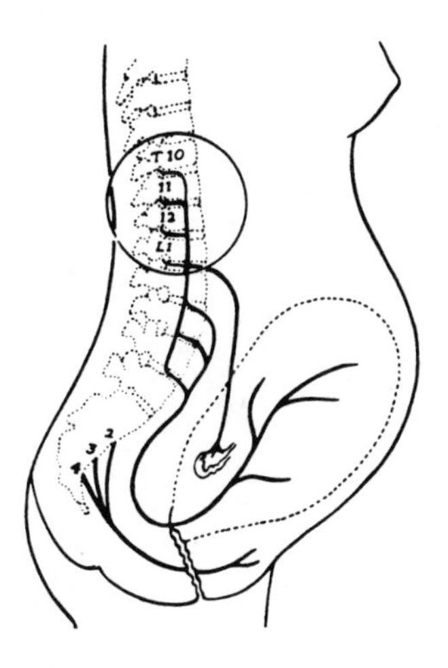

FIG C–1.

Neurology of labor pain; mechanisms and pathways for peripheral parturition pain. *First stage:* Stretching and possible tearing of the cervix and contraction and distention of the uterus. Early and mild pain sensations are transmitted to the 11th and 12th thoracic spinal cord segments. When the pain becomes more intense the two adjacent segments become involved (to total L1 to T10). The cervix has the same pain pathways as the body of the uterus. *Second stage:* Distention, stretching, and tearing of fascia, skin, and subcutaneous tissues of the perineum. Transmitted via the pudendal nerve to the sacral segments S2, S3, and S4. *Other (less important) factors:* (1) Traction on the adnexa and parietal peritoneum; (2) distention and stretching of the bladder, urethra, and rectum; (3) pressure on, and stretching of, nerve roots of the lumbosacral plexus (above three sources of pain are transmitted via various nerves to L2 to S4 spinal segments; and (4) reflex muscle spasm of muscle groups innervated by the same spinal segments as the uterus T11 to T12 (and to lesser extent T10, L1). Note that the dermatomes that correspond to these levels are in the lower back. (Modified from Bonica JJ: *Obstetric Analgesia and Anesthesia*. Amsterdam, World Federation of Societies of Anaesthesiologists, 1980, p 45. As published in Main DM, Main EK: *Obstetrics and Gynecology. A Pocket Reference*. St Louis, Mosby–Year Book, 1984. Used by permission.)

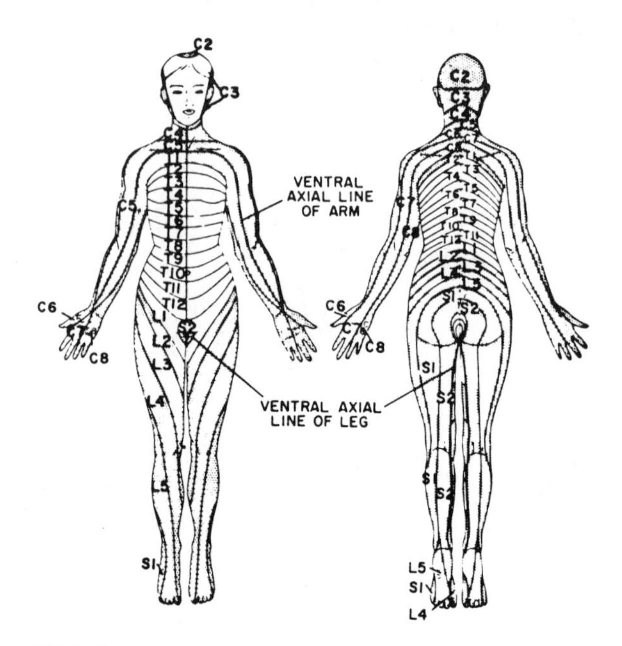

FIG C–2.

Dermatomes. Knowledge of the spinal dermatomes is helpful in determining levels of epidural or spinal anesthesia. There are two dermatomal charts in common use today that are in general agreement as to the levels on the trunk (a good guidepost is that the umbilicus = T10), but disagree markedly on the distribution on the limbs. This (perhaps more widely used) chart shows the dermatomes extending as strips nearly the length of the limb. The alternative chart (Forester) indicates a more patchy distribution. The relative clinical correctness is not resolved. There is a clear mistake on the above chart, however, in that C5 and T1 do not extend significantly onto the thorax; rather, C3 and C4 supply this area. (From Keegan JJ, Garrett FD: *Anat Rec* 1948; 102:409. Used by permission.)

TABLE C–1.
Characteristics of Local Anesthetics*

Anesthetic	Class	Use	Onset	Duration (min)	Single Maximum Dose (mg)
Low Potency					
Procaine (Novocain, Winthrop)	Ester	Local	Slow	60–90	800† 1,000‡
Intermediate Potency					
Chloroprocaine HCl (Nesacaine, Astra)	Ester	Local, nerve block, epidural	Fast	30–90	800† 1,000‡
Lidocaine (Xylocaine, Astra)	Amide	Local, nerve block, epidural, spinal	Fast	90–200	300† 500‡
Mepivacaine (Carbocaine, Winthrop)	Amide	Local, nerve block, epidural	Fast	120–240	400
High Potency					
Tetracaine (Pontocaine, Winthrop)	Ester	Spinal	Slow	180–600	200
Bupivacaine (Marcaine, Winthrop; Sensorcaine, Astra)	Amide	Local, nerve block, epidural, spinal	Slow	180–600	175† 225‡
Etidocaine (Duranest, Astra)	Amide	Nerve block, epidural	Fast	180–600	300† 400‡
Dibucaine (Nupercaine, Ciba)	Amide	Spinal	Slow	180–240	10
Prilocaine (Citanest, Astra	Amide	Nerve block, epidural	Fast	120–240	600

*From Zatuchni GI, Slupik R: *Obstetrics and Gynecology Drug Handbook*. St Louis, Mosby–Year Book, p 17. Used by permission.
†Without epinephrine.
‡With epinephrine.

TABLE C–2.
Systemic Analgesia in Labor*

A. ***Narcotics***[1, 2]

Meperidine (Demerol) has achieved the widest popularity for systemic analgesia during labor. It appears to produce less nausea and emesis than morphine in parturients and may produce slightly less neonatal depression (this difference is probably minor, if existent, with the smaller doses now in common use).

Dose

Currently recommended doses in labor include:

IM 50–100 mg

IV 25–40 mg

Timing for repetitive doses remains controversial. **(Morphine** doses are 1/10 the above doses.)

Metabolism of meperidine is complex with at least two active metabolites. Additionally there appear to be three types of degradation patterns with quite different time courses. This could account for some of the individual variation both in analgesic effects and neonatal depression.

Side effects

It should be stressed that when equi-analgesic doses are used all narcotics produce similar side effects. Each newly introduced drug's claim for reduced side effects has not held up with clinical usage. The only possible exception may be butorphanol (Stadol) which, apparently, has different properties than the classic narcotics. The risks of respiratory depression with Stadol in mother or infant do not seem to increase with increasing doses.[3] (Usual dosage range: 1 mg IV, 1–2 mg IM.) Further investigation needs to be performed with this new agent.

Newborn depression: Peak depressant effect on the newborn is seen during the second and third hour after administration. Little or no significant depression is noted if the infant is born within the first hour after dosage or after the fourth hour. Some investigators have found that total administered dose also correlates with neonatal effects. Fetal CNS depression is also commonly seen, usually manifested as loss of short and long term beat-to-beat variability. Another FHT abnormality reported, particularly after alphaprodine (Nisentil) administration, is the sinusoidal pattern.

Signs of narcotic depression in the newborn include:

1. Central respiratory depression
2. Miosis (pupillary constriction)
3. Absence of reflexes
4. Hypotonia

Agent of choice for reversal is **naloxone** (Narcan): 0.01 mg/kg IM (acts in 3–5 min) or IV (acts in 30–90 sec).

Effects on labor: Narcotics may slow the progress of labor if given during latent phase or if the dose is excessive (transiently such an effect can be seen with rapid IV injection of an optimal dose).

Maternal side effects: Respiratory depression and orthostatic hypotension are the most serious problems and need to be watched for carefully. They are rarely seen in this setting unless dosage guidelines are exceeded.

B. ***Diazepam (Valium)***

Diazepam has been used commonly during labor especially in Europe. Its use in the U.S. has been restricted because of concern for the side effects listed below. Kinetics after an IM injection include: a maternal peak in 30 min; fetal peak in 60 min, after which point fetal levels always exceed maternal levels. Immature fetal liver enzymes prevent complete metabolism. Common fetal/newborn side effects:

1. Loss of fetal heart rate variability
2. Respiratory depression
3. Hypotonia
4. Decreased suck reflex
5. Decreased temperature control
6. Apnea

These effects are usually seen after doses of 20 mg or more and are uncommon with doses less than 10 mg. It should be remembered that these side effects cannot be reversed with naloxone.

C. ***Beneficial effects of maternal systemic analgesic***

While most recent literature has focused on the potential for ill effects on the newborn, a review by Myers and Myers[4] emphasized the possibility for systemic analgesia to prevent or reduce asphyxia. Some of the proposed mechanisms included: Decreasing maternal sympathetic activity and improving uterine blood flow, and depressing fetal brain metabolism leading to increasing fetal tolerance to asphyxia.

Selected references:

1. Fishburne JI: Systemic analgesia during labor. *Clin Perinatol* 1982; 9:29. (The entire issue, February 1982, is devoted to obstetric anesthesia and analgesia.)
2. Bonica JS: *Principles and Practice of Obstetric Anesthesia.* Philadelphia, FA Davis, 1967.
3. Quilligan EJ, Keegan KA, Donahue MJ: Double blind comparison of intravenously injected butorphanol and meperidine in parturients. *Int J Gynecol Obstet* 1980; 18:363.
4. Myers RE, Myers SE: Use of sedative, analgesic, and anesthetic drugs during labor and delivery: Bane or boon? *Am J Obstet Gynecol* 1979; 133:83.

*From Main DM, Main EK: *Obstetrics and Gynecology. A Pocket Reference.* St Louis, Mosby–Year Book, 1984. Used by permission.

FETAL PHYSIOLOGY

APPENDIX D: CHROMOSOMAL ABNORMALITIES

TABLE D–1.

Estimates of Rates per Thousand of Chromosome Abnormalities in Live Births by Single-Year Interval*

Maternal Age	Down's Syndrome	Edwards Syndrome (Trisomy 18)	Patau Syndrome (Trisomy 13)	XXY	XYY	Turner Syndrome Genotype	Other Clinically Significant Abnormality†	Total‡
<15	1.0§	<0.1§	<0.1–0.1	0.4	0.5	<0.1	0.2	2.2
15	1.0§	<0.1§	<0.1–0.1	0.4	0.5	<0.1	0.2	2.2
16	0.9§	<0.1§	<0.1–0.1	0.4	0.5	<0.1	0.2	2.1
17	0.8§	<0.1§	<0.1–0.1	0.4	0.5	<0.1	0.2	2.0
18	0.7§	<0.1§	<0.1–0.1	0.4	0.5	<0.1	0.2	1.9
19	0.6§	<0.1§	<0.1–0.1	0.4	0.5	<0.1	0.2	1.8
20	0.5–0.7	<0.1–0.1	<0.1–0.1	0.4	0.5	<0.1	0.2	1.9
21	0.5–0.7	<0.1–0.1	<0.1–0.1	0.4	0.5	<0.1	0.2	1.9
22	0.6–0.8	<0.1–0.1	<0.1–0.1	0.4	0.5	<0.1	0.2	2.0
23	0.6–0.8	<0.1–0.1	<0.1–0.1	0.4	0.5	<0.1	0.2	2.0
24	0.7–0.9	0.1–0.1	<0.1–0.1	0.4	0.5	<0.1	0.2	2.1
25	0.7–0.9	0.1–0.1	<0.1–0.1	0.4	0.5	<0.1	0.2	2.1
26	0.7–1.0	0.1–0.1	<0.1–0.1	0.4	0.5	<0.1	0.2	2.1
27	0.8–1.0	0.1–0.2	<0.1–0.1	0.4	0.5	<0.1	0.2	2.2
28	0.8–1.1	0.1–0.2	<0.1–0.2	0.4	0.5	<0.1	0.2	2.3
29	0.8–1.2	0.1–0.2	<0.1–0.2	0.5	0.5	<0.1	0.2	2.4
30	0.9–1.2	0.1–0.2	<0.1–0.2	0.5	0.5	<0.1	0.2	2.6
31	0.9–1.3	0.1–0.2	<0.1–0.2	0.5	0.5	<0.1	0.2	2.6

32	1.1–1.5	0.1–0.2	0.1–0.2	0.6	0.5	<0.1	0.2	3.1
33	1.4–1.9	0.1–0.3	0.1–0.2	0.7	0.5	<0.1	0.2	3.5
34	1.9–2.4	0.2–0.4	0.1–0.3	0.7	0.5	<0.1	0.2	4.1
35	2.5–3.9	0.3–0.5	0.2–0.3	0.9	0.5	<0.1	0.3	5.6
36	3.2–5.0	0.3–0.6	0.2–0.4	1.0	0.5	<0.1	0.3	6.7
37	4.1–6.4	0.4–0.7	0.2–0.5	1.1	0.5	<0.1	0.3	8.1
38	5.2–8.1	0.5–0.9	0.3–0.7	1.3	0.5	<0.1	0.3	9.5
39	6.6–10.5	0.7–1.2	0.4–0.8	1.5	0.5	<0.1	0.3	12.4
40	8.5–13.7	0.9–1.6	0.5–1.1	1.8	0.5	<0.1	0.3	15.8
41	10.8–17.9	1.2–2.1	0.6–1.4	2.2	0.5	<0.1	0.3	20.5
42	13.8–23.4	1.4–2.7	0.7–1.8	2.7	0.5	<0.1	0.3	25.5
43	17.6–30.6	1.8–3.5	0.9–2.4	3.3	0.5	<0.1	0.3	32.6
44	22.5–40.0	2.3–4.6	1.2–3.1	4.1	0.5	<0.1	0.3	41.8
45	28.7–52.3	2.9–6.0	1.5–4.1	5.1	0.5	<0.1	0.3	53.7
46	36.6–68.3	3.7–7.9	1.9–5.3	6.4	0.5	<0.1	0.3	68.9
47	46.6–89.3	4.7–10.3	2.4–6.9	8.2	0.5	<0.1	0.3	89.1
48	59.5–116.8	6.0–13.5	3.0–9.0	10.6	0.5	<0.1	0.3	115.0
49	75.8–152.7	7.6–17.6	3.8–11.8	13.8	0.5	<0.1	0.3	149.3

*From Hook EB: *Obstet Gynecol* 1981; 58:282. As published in Main DM, Main EK: *Obstetrics and Gynecology. A Pocket Reference.* St Louis, Mosby–Year Book, 1984. Used by permission.

†XXX is excluded.

‡Calculation of the total at each age assumes rate for autosomal aneuploidies is at the midpoints of the ranges given.

§No range may be constructed for those under 20 years by the same methods as for those 20 and over. These age-related risk estimates are for women who present with no other risk factor except age. They are derived from multiple regression studies of *live births* of chromosomally abnormal infants.

TABLE E–1.

Estimated Dose to Uterus From Extraabdominal Examinations* (Fluoroscopic Dose Excluded)*

Examination	Estimated Mean Dose (mrad/Examination)			Reported Range‖
	BRH†	ICRP‡	UNSCEAR§	
Dental		<10	0.06	0.03–0.1
Head-cervical spine	<0.5	<10	<10	<0.5–3.0
Extremities	<0.5	<10	<10	<0.5–18.0
Shoulder	<0.5	<10		<0.5–3.0
Thoracic spine	11	<10		<10–55
Chest (radiographic)	1		2	0.2–43
Chest (photofluorographic)	3	<10	3	0.9–40
Mammography			<10	
Femur (distal)		50	1	1–50
Upper gastrointestinal series	171	150		5–1,230
Cholecystography	78	150	120	14–1,600
Cholngiography				
Lumbar spine	990		560	27–3,970
Lumbosacral spine		550	470	100–2,440
Pelvis	290	340	320	55–2,190
Hips and femur (proximal)	170	690	330	73–1,370

Urography, intravenous, or		960	810	70–5,480
retrograde pyleogram	810	1,100	715	120–5,480
Urethrocystography		2,060		275–4,110
Lower gastrointestinal tract (barium enema)	1,240	1,100	1,200	28–12,600
Abdomen	300	690	290	25–1,920
Abdomen (obstetric)		1,370 (fetal)	410	150–2,200
Pelvimetry		5,480	850	220–5,480
Hysterosalpingography		1,650	1,740	270–9,180

*Adapted from National Council on Radiation Protection and Measurements (NCRP), 1977; and Wagner LK, Lester RG, Saldana LR: *Exposure of the Pregnant Patient to Diagnostic Radiations: A Guide to Medical Management.* Philadelphia, JP Lippincott, 1985, p 53. All values are for radiography only (no fluoroscopy). Doses listed for lower abdominal studies are 37% higher than those in NCRP (1977).

†Bureau of Radiological Health (BRH) (1976).

‡International Commission of Radiological Protection (CRP) (1970).

§United Nations Scientific Committee on the Effects of Atomic Radiation (UNSCEAR) (1972).

‖Includes BRH (1976), ICRP (1970), UNSCEAR (1972), and Lindell and Dobson (1961).

APPENDIX E: DIAGNOSTIC RADIOLOGY AND THE FETUS

I. Diagnostic Radiologic Procedures and Level of Fetal Radiation Exposure

A. Radiographs

1. **X-ray** (Table E–1, previous pages).
2. **Computed Tomography.** The fetal exposure with this radiologic modality has been difficult to determine. The following is a rough guide to estimated fetal dosage (Table E–2).

B. Magnetic Resonance Imaging. No radiation is used with this form of scanning.

C. Occupational Exposure. The National Council of Radiation Protection and Measurement recommends that mothers facing occupational radiation exposure not be exposed to more than 0.5 rads throughout their pregnancy.

II. Effects of Radiation on the Fetus

A. Time of Exposure

1. Fetal radiation exposure soon after conception will result either in abortion or an unaffected fetus.
2. Fetal radiation exposure between 8 and 15 weeks' gestation demonstrates a linear relationship between the absorbed fetal dose and severe mental retardation. The risk has been estimated at 0.4% per rad (*Br J Radiol* 1984; 57:409–414; quoted in Columbia Presbyterian draft policy concerning occupationally exposed women who are or

TABLE E–2.
Estimated Average Fetal Dose per Diagnostic Radiologic Examination: Computed Tomography

Examination	Typical Dose to Fetus
Head scan	Insignificant
Extremity	Insignificant
Chest	Insignificant to low
Abdominal with or without contrast	Below 10 rads*

*Varies with fetal proximity to the area being studied.

could be pregnant. Columbia cites this as a follow-up study of children born to mothers who received pelvic irradiation in Hiroshima and Nagasaki. According to one source [Harrison citation], microcephaly showed a statistical increase at doses at or above 10–19 rads, small stature 25 rads, and mental retardation 50 rads. This is far above current radiographic dosages.) (Table E–3)

B. Exposure Dose

1. >50 rads (Grey). At this level of fetal exposure a significant chance of an embryopathic event is present.
2. >15 rads (Grey). The rise of malformations is significantly increased above control levels. Only exposures above this level warrant consideration of pregnancy termination.
3. ≤10 rads (grey). Many authors claim never to have seen congenital defects at this dose level. However, low levels of intrauterine radiation (1–3 rads) (Harrison) may be associated with a small increase in the risk (1.5–2.0×) of leukemia and of chromosomal abnormalities in germ cells, although this is controversial. (For example, in one large study the control risk of leukemia = 1/2,880; the risk of those exposed to pelvimetry = 1/2,000.*)
4. Intrauterine growth retardation and central nervous system abnormalities (microcephaly, cerebral and cerebellar hypoplasia) may be seen throughout gestation with *therapeutic* doses of radiation. It is unlikely that a major anomaly in an infant is due to radiation if fetal growth or the CNS has not been affected.*
5. All pregnant women exposed to radiation must be made aware of the possible long-term effects of this exposure.

III. Conversion of Radiologic Units

A. A **roentgen** (R) is a measure of the quantity of X or gamma ionizing radiation in the air.

B. The **radiation absorbed dose** (rad) is a measure of the energy absorbed by tissue from ionizing radiation equivalent to 100 ergs of energy/gram. For practical purposes, the R and the rad are equivalent.

*Main DM, Main EK: *Obstetrics and Gynecology. A Pocket Reference*. St Louis, Mosby–Year Book, 1984. Modified from an excellent review on the subject: Brent RI. Irradiation in pregnancy, in Sciarra J (ed): *Gynecology and Obstetrics, vol 2*. Hagerstown, Md, Harper & Row, 1979, chap 19.

TABLE E–3.

Summary of Effects of Diagnostic Levels of Radiation (0–25 rads) on the Unborn*†

Weeks Post-conception		Gestation Stage	Effect				
			Prenatal Death	Small Head Size (SHS)	Severe Mental Retardation (SMR)	Other Malformation	Childhood Cancer
1st Trimester	0–	Preimplantation	Possible radiation-induced resorption	None established for humans at diagnostic levels	None established for humans at diagnostic levels	None established for humans at diagnostic levels	Higher risk period
	2–	Major organogenesis	None established for humans at diagnostic levels	Incidence of 1% per rad at Hiroshima, but causal nature of radiation is uncertain		Animal data suggest this is most sensitive stage, but none established for humans at diagnostic levels	
	6–						

	Weeks						
2nd and 3rd Trimester	8–	Synaptogenesis Rapid neuron development and migration			SMR at 0.4% per rad from A-bomb, but radiation may not have been sole cause of this effect	None established for humans at diagnostic levels	Lesser risk period
	15–						
	16–			None established for humans at diagnostic levels	None established for humans at diagnostic levels		
	38–						

*Adapted from Wagner LK, Lester RG, Saldana LR: *Exposure of the Pregnant Patient to Diagnostic Radiations. A Guide to Medical Management.* Philadelphia, JP Lippincott, 1985, p 70.

†Effects from placental transfer of radionuclides are not included.

C. A **rem** is the dose in rads multiplied by the quality factor (the quality factor equals 1 for the radiations encountered with x- and gamma rays, electrons and photons). This unit allows radiologists to describe the observation that some forms of radiation, such as neutrons, may produce a greater biological effect per dose of absorbed energy.

D. The rad and the rem are commonly used terminology in the United States. Internationally, they are comparable to the Grey and the Sievert in the following manner:

100 rads = 1 Grey (Gy)
100 rems = 1 Sievert (Sv)

BIBLIOGRAPHY

Harrison JA: Radiation in pregnancy, in Goldstein AI: *Advances in Perinatal Medicine*. New York, Symposia Specialists Medical Books, 1977, pp 29–39.

Howland WJ (ed): *Radiation Biology Syllabus and Questions for Diagnostic Radiology Residents*. Oak Brook, IL, Radiological Society of North America, 1982.

Main DM, Main EK: *Obstetrics and Gynecology. A Pocket Reference*. St Louis, Mosby–Year Book, 1984.

Medical Radiation Exposure of Pregnant and Potentially Pregnant Women. NCRP Report No. 54. National Council on Radiation Protection and Measurements, Bethesda, Md, May 1, 1985.

Mossman KL, Hill LT: Radiation risks in pregnancy. *Obstet Gynecol* 1982; 60:237–242.

Policy Concerning Occupationally Exposed Women Who Are or Could Be Pregnant (Draft). New York, Columbia Presbyterian Medical Center, 1990.

APPENDIX F: FETAL CIRCULATION*

TABLE F–1.

Fetal Structure	From/To	Adult Remnant
1. Umbilical vein	Umbilicus/ductus venosus	Ligamentum teres hepatitis
2. Ductus venosus	Umbilical vein/inferior vena cava (bypasses liver)	Ligamentum venosum
3. Foramen ovale	Right atrium/left atrium	Closed atrial wall
4. Ductus arteriosus	Pulmonary artery/descending aorta	Ligamentum arteriosum
5. Umbilical artery	Common iliac artery/umbilicus	1. Superior vesicle arteries 2. Lateral vesicoumbilical ligaments

*From Gabbe SG, Niebyl JR, Simpson JL: *Obstetrics: Normal and Problem Pregnancies.* New York, Churchill Livingstone, 1986. Used by permission.

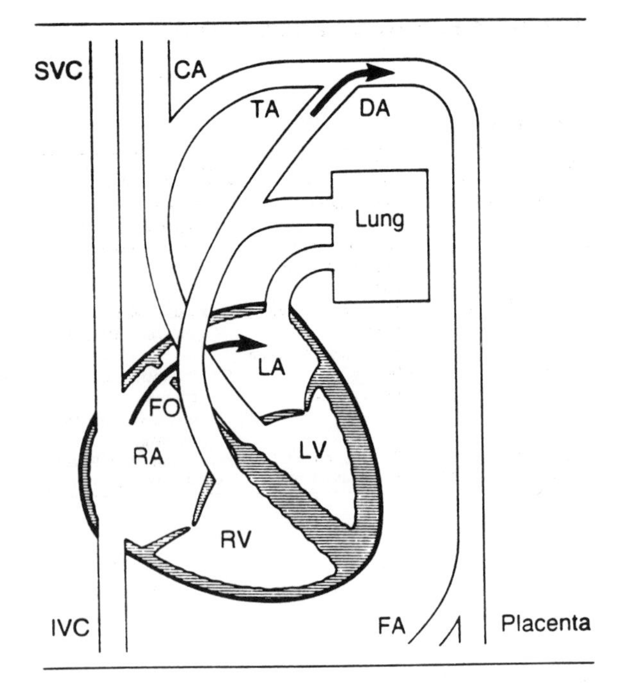

FIG F–1.
Anatomy of fetal heart and central shunts. *SVC* = superior vena cava; *CA* = carotid artery; *TA* = thoracic aorta; *DA* = ductus arteriosus; *RA* = right atrium; *FO* = foramen ovale; *LA* = left atrium; *RV* = right ventricle; *LV* = left ventricle; *IVC* = inferior vena cava; *FA* = femoral artery. (From Anderson DF, Bissonnette JM, Faber JJ, et al: *Am J Physiol* 1981; 241 (*Heart Circ Physiol* 10):H60. Used by permission.)

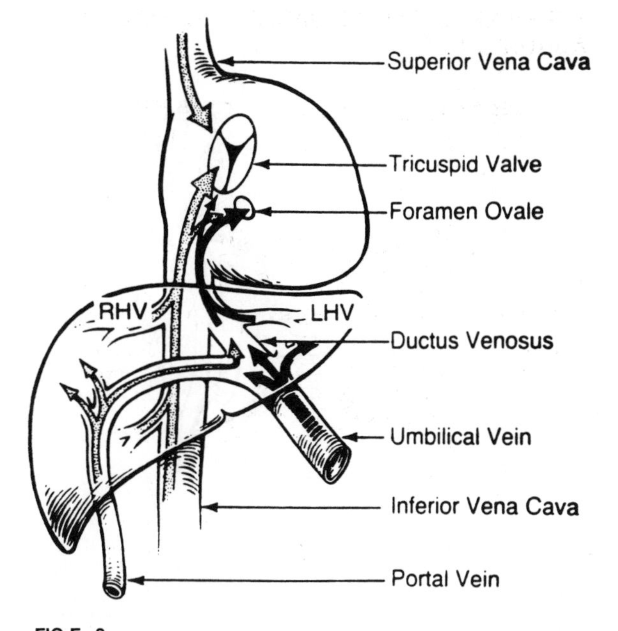

FIG F–2.
Anatomy of the umbilical and hepatic circulation. *RHV* = right hepatic vein; *LHV* = left hepatic vein. (From Rudolph AM: *Hepatology* 1983; 3:254. Used by permission.)

APPENDIX G: BLOOD GASES—NORMAL AND ABNORMAL

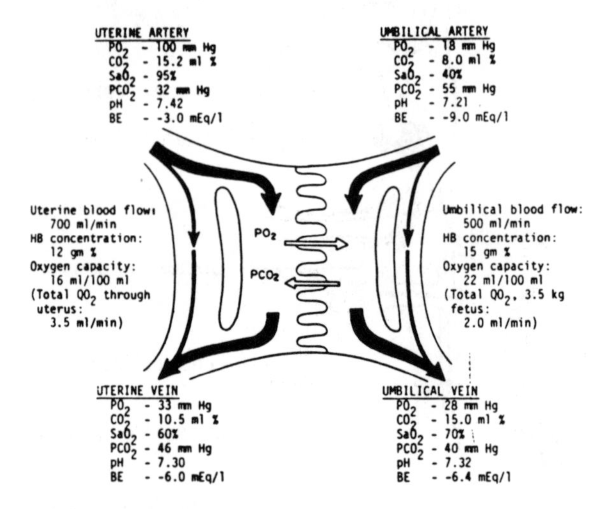

FIG G–1.

Placental transfer of oxygen and carbon dioxide. These data represent a synthesis of estimations from clinical material and extrapolations from sheep models. (From Bonica JJ: *Obstetric Analgesia and Anesthesia,* ed 2. Amsterdam, World Federation of Societies of Anesthesiologists, 1980, p 29. Used by permission.)

TABLE G–1.
Definitions

Acidemia:	Increased concentration of hydrogen ions in the blood
Acidosis:	A pathologic condition marked by an increased concentration of hydrogen ions in tissue
Hypoxemia:	Decreased oxygen content in blood
Hypoxia:	A pathologic condition marked by a decreased level of oxygen in tissue
Asphyxia:	Hypoxia and metabolic acidosis

TABLE G–2.
Classification of Fetal or Newborn Acidemia*, †

Acidemia Type	pCO_2 (mm Hg)	HCO_3^- (mEq/L)	Base Deficit (mEq/L)‡
Respiratory	High (>65)	Normal (≥22)	Normal (−6.4 ± 1.9)
Metabolic	Normal (<65)	Low (≤17)	High (−15.9 ± 2.8)
Mixed	High (≥65)	Low (≤17)	High (−9.6 ± 2.5)

*From *Assessment of Fetal and Newborn Acid-Base Status.* ACOG Technical Bulletin No. 127, April 1989. Used by permission.
†Umbilical artery pH less than 7.20.
‡Means ± standard deviations are given in parentheses.

TABLE G–3.
Normal Values for Umbilical Cord Blood*, †

Cord Blood	pH	pCO_2 (mm Hg)	pO_2 (mm Hg)	Bicarbonate (mEq/L)
Arterial	7.28 ± 0.05	49.2 ± 8.4	18.0 ± 6.2	22.3 ± 2.5
	(7.15 – 7.43)	(31.1 – 74.3)	(3.8 – 33.8)	(13.3 – 27.5)
Venous	7.35 ± 0.05	38.2 ± 5.6	29.2 ± 5.9	20.4 ± 2.1
	(7.24 – 7.49)	(23.2 – 49.2)	(15.4 – 48.2)	(15.9 – 24.7)

*From *Assessment of Fetal and Newborn Acid-Base Status.* ACOG Technical Bulletin No. 127, April 1989. Used by permission.
†Results are for 146 newborns after uncomplicated labor and vaginal delivery at 37–42 weeks of gestation. Values are mean ± standard deviation; ranges are given in parentheses (Yeomans ER, Hauth JC, Gilstrap LC III, et al: Umbilical cord pH, PCO_2 and bicarbonate following uncomplicated term vaginal deliveries. *Am J Obstet Gynecol* 1985; 15:798–800).

APPENDIX H: ULTRASOUND EVALUATION: FETAL GROWTH

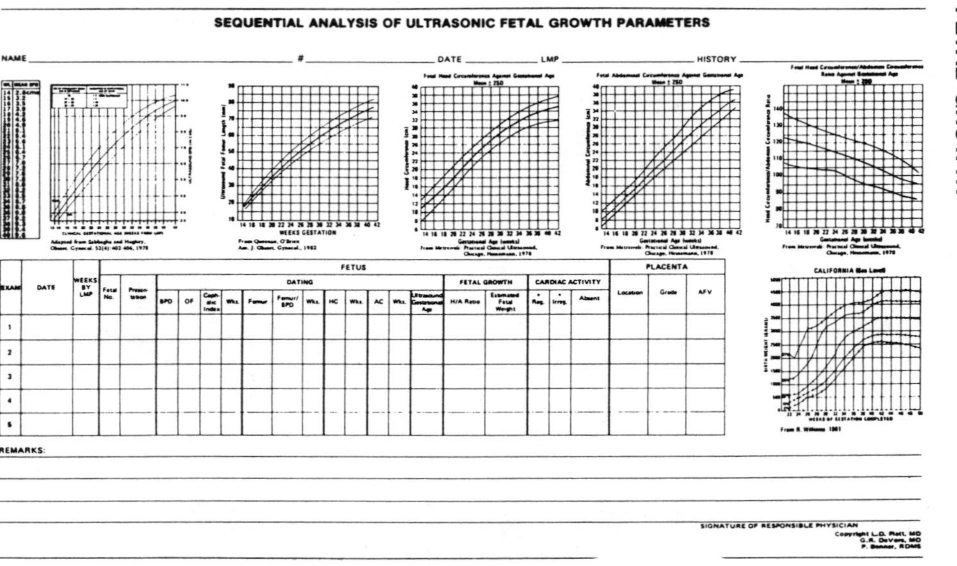

SEQUENTIAL ANALYSIS OF ULTRASONIC FETAL GROWTH PARAMETERS

NAME ______________ # ______________ DATE ______________ LMP ______________ HISTORY ______________

EXAM	DATE	WEEKS BY LMP	FETUS																			PLACENTA		
					DATING												FETAL GROWTH		CARDIAC ACTIVITY					
			Fetal No.	Presentation	BPD	OF	Cephalic Index	Wks.	Femur	Femur/BPD	Wks.	HC	Wks.	AC	Wks.	Ultrasound Gestational Age	H/A Ratio	Estimated Fetal Weight	+ Reg.	+ Irreg.	Absent	Location	Grade	AFV
1																								
2																								
3																								
4																								
5																								

REMARKS:

SIGNATURE OF RESPONSIBLE PHYSICIAN

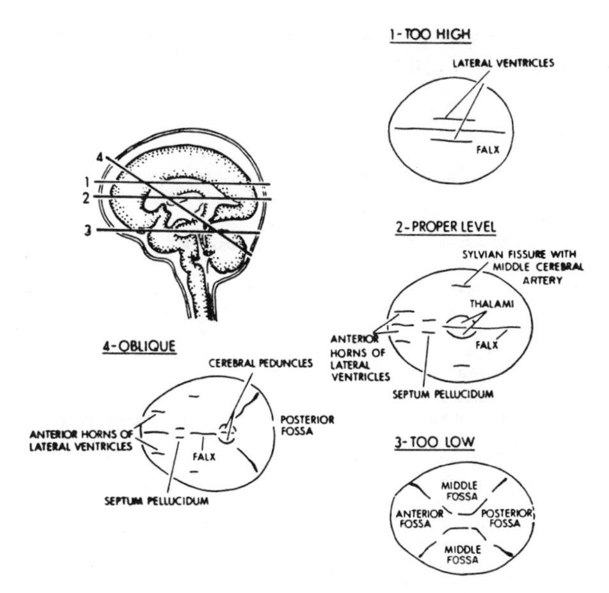

FIG H–2.
Landmarks for obtaining a proper biparietal diameter. These drawings demonstrate the landmarks seen when placing the ultrasound transducer in too high, correct, too low, or oblique positions. (Adapted from materials developed by J. P. Crane, Washington University, St Louis, Mo. As published in Main DM, Main EK: *Obstetrics and Gynecology. A Pocket Reference*. St Louis, Mosby–Year Book, 1984. Used by permission.)

FIG H–1.
Sequential analysis of ultrasonic fetal growth parameters. (From Gabbe SG, Niebyl JR, Simpson JL. *Obstetrics: Normal and Problem Pregnancies*. New York, Churchill Livingstone, 1986. Used by permission.)

APPENDIX I: ULTRASOUND EVALUATION: AMNIOTIC FLUID VOLUME

TABLE I–1.
Oligohydramnios[1–4,*]

Definition

<200 ml amniotic fluid at term.

Ultrasound definition: Amniotic fluid index (AFI) less than 5 cm.

Diagnosis

1. Antenatal diagnosis is clinically difficult. It has been suggested that oligohydramnios can be diagnosed by ultrasound when the largest pocket of amniotic fluid measures less than 1 cm in its broadest diameter.[1]
2. Presence of amnion nodosum on placenta at delivery is highly correlated with oligohydramnios

Clinical associations

1. Fetal malformations, particularly renal agenesis, polycystic kidneys, ureteral and urethral obstruction and agenesis of the penis.
2. Extramembranous pregnancies.
3. Prolonged leakage of amniotic fluid.
4. Intrauterine growth retardation, particularly secondary to pregnancy-induced hypertension and other conditions that induce placental insufficiency.
5. Postmaturity syndrome.

Fetal anomalies associated with prolonged oligohydramnios

(Usually after a minimum 3 wk of oligohydramnios.[2–4]

1. Potter's facies: increased space between eyes, prominent fold that arises from inner canthus and sweeps downward and laterally below the eyes, nasal flattening, excessive recession of the chin, enlarged and lowset ears.
2. Pulmonary hypoplasia and insufficiency.
3. Limb malpositions such as clubbed feet.
4. Fetal growth retardation.

Selected references:

1. Manning FA, Hill LM, Platt LD: Qualitative amniotic fluid volume determination by ultrasound: Antepartum detection of intrauterine growth retardation, *Am J Obstet Gynecol* 1981; 139:254.
2. Potter EL: Bilateral renal agenesis, *J Pediatr* 1946; 29:68.
3. Bain AD, Smith II, Gauld IK: Newborn after prolonged leakage of liquor amnii, *Br Med J* 1964; 2:598.
4. Perlman M, Williams I, Hirsch M: Neonatal pulmonary hypoplasia after prolonged leakage of amniotic fluid, *Arch Dis Child* 1976; 51:349.

*Modified from Main DM, Main EK: *Obstetrics and Gynecology. A Pocket Reference.* St Louis, Mosby–Year Book, 1984. Used by permission.

TABLE I–2.
Incidence of Polyhydramnios and Associated Conditions*

	Incidence†	
	No.	%
Total deliveries	86,301	100.00
Polyhydramnios‡	358	0.41
Associated conditions		
Diabetes	88	24.6
Erythroblastosis fetalis	41	11.5
Multiple gestation	33	9.2
Congenital malformations§	72	20.1
Idiopathic	124	34.6
Total	358	100.0

*From Main DM, Main EK: *Obstetrics and Gynecology. A Pocket Reference.* St Louis, Mosby–Year Book, 1984. Used by permission.

†Data from Queenan JT, Gadow EC: *Am J Obstet Gynecol* 1970; 108:349. Based on a 20-year retrospective study in one institution (1948–1967). Polyhydramnios defined as ≥2,000 ml amniotic fluid, 1.7% acute, 98.3 chronic.

‡**Polyhydramnios** clinical definition: ≥ 2,000 mL amniotic fluid.
Polyhydramnios, ultrasound definition: Amniotic fluid index greater than 25 cm or a single pocket greater than 8 cm.

§Approximately 50% of the congenital anomalies will involve the CNS, 20% the GI tract, and 20% the heart. (From Murray SR: *Am J Obstet Gynecol* 1964; 88:65; Jacoby HE, Charles D: *Am J Obstet Gynecol* 1966; 94:110.)

APPENDIX J: ULTRASOUND EVALUATION: PLACENTAL GRADING

The placenta may be assessed by ultrasound evaluation. As the placenta matures, its ultrasonic appearance changes. Table J–1 and Fig J–1 illustrate the commonly used placental grading system.

TABLE J–1.
Summary of Placental Grading*

	Placental Grade			
Section of Placenta	0	1	2	3
Chorionic plate	Straight and well defined	Subtle undulations	Indentations extending into placenta but not to basal layer	Indentations communicating with basal layer
Placental substance	Homogeneous	Few scattered EGAs	Linear echogenic densities (commalike densities)	Circular densities with echo-spared areas in center; large, irregular densities casting acoustic shadows
Basal layer	No densities	No densities	Linear arrangement of small EGAs (basal stippling)	Large and somewhat confluent basal EGAs; can create acoustic shadows

*From Gabbe SG, Niebl JR, Simpson JL. *Obstetrics: Normal and Problem Pregnancies.* New York, Churchill Livingstone, 1986. Used by permission.
EGA = echogenic areas.
Grannum P, Berkowitz R, Hobbins J: The ultrasonic changes in the maturing placenta and their relation to fetal pulmonic maturity. *Am J Obstet Gynecol* 1979; 133:915.

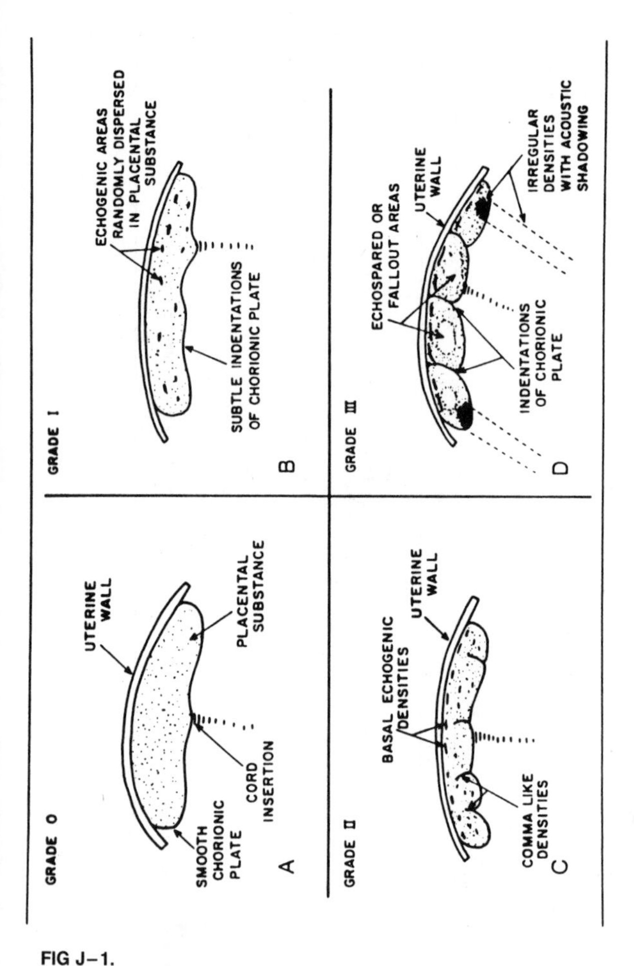

FIG J–1.
The four stages of placental maturation based on the appearance of the basal and chorionic plate of the placenta and the placental substance. (From Grannum PAT, Berkowitz RL, Hobbins JC: *Am J Obstet Gynecol* 1979; 133:915. Used by permission.)

APPENDIX K: INTRAPARTUM FETAL HEART RATE MONITORING

TABLE K–1.

Grading of Late Decelerations*

Definition

The onset of the deceleration is usually more than 30 sec after the onset of the contraction with the nadir of the deceleration following the peak of the contraction. The descent from and return to baseline are smooth and gradual.

Grades	*Mild*	*Moderate*	*Severe*
Amplitude of drop in FHTs	<15 bpm	15–45 bpm	>45 bpm

All lates must be considered significant and potentially ominous *regardless of* severity grade. Associated lack of variability and tachycardia are further predictors of fetal acidosis.

*From Kubli FW, et al: *Am J Obstet Gynecol* 1969; 104:1190. As published in Main DM, Main EK: *Obstetrics and Gynecology. A Pocket Reference*. St Louis, Mosby–Year Book, 1984. Used by permission.

FHTs = fetal heart tones.

TABLE K–2.

Fetal Scalp pH in Relation to Fetal Heart Rate Patterns* †

FHT Pattern	Scalp pH	Number of Samples
No deceleration	7.30 ± 0.042	71
Early deceleration	7.30 ± 0.041	16
Variable deceleration (mild)	7.29 ± 0.046	42
Variable deceleration (moderate)	7.26 ± 0.044	35
Late deceleration (mild)	7.22 ± 0.060	27
Late deceleration (moderate)	7.21 ± 0.054	7
Variable deceleration (severe)	7.15 ± 0.069	10
Late deceleration (severe)	7.12 ± 0.066	10

*Adapted from Kubli FW, et al: *Am J Obstet Gynecol* 1969; 104:1190. As published in Main DM, Main EK: *Obstetrics and Gynecology. A Pocket Reference.* St Louis, Mosby–Year Book, 1984. Used by permission.

†FHT = fetal heart tone.

TABLE K–3.
Causes of Decreased Fetal Heart Rate Variability[1–3, *]

Hypoxia/acidosis	Congenital anomalies
Drugs (see below)	Extreme prematurity
Fetal sleep cycles	Fetal tachycardia

Examples of Drugs Causing Decreased Fetal Heart Rate Variability

1. CNS depressants
   - Analgesic/narcotics
     - Demerol
     - Nisentil
     - Morphine
   - Barbiturates
     - Phenobarbital
     - Secobarbital
   - Tranquilizers
     - Diazepam
   - Phenothiazines
     - Phenergan
   - Sedatives/antihistamines
     - Vistaril/Atarax
2. Parasympatholitics
   - Atropine
   - Scopolamine
3. General anesthetics
4. Magnesium sulfate appears *not* to decrease variability[2]

Selected references:

1. Petrie RH, et al: The effects of drugs on fetal heart rate variability, *Am J Obstet Gynecol* 1978; 130:294.
2. Stallworth JC, Yeh S, Petrie RH: The effect of magnesium sulfate on fetal heart rate variability and uterine activity. *Am J Obstet Gynecol* 1981; 140:702.
3. Freeman RK, Garite TJ: *Fetal Heart Rate Monitoring.* Baltimore, Williams & Wilkins, 1981.

*From Main DM, Main EK: *Obstetrics and Gynecology. A Pocket Reference.* St Louis, Mosby–Year Book, 1984. Used by permission.

TABLE K–4.
Causes of Fetal Bradycardia[1–4, *]

1. Physiologic (not associated with fetal acidosis)
   a. 100–120 bpm with good variability during the first stage of labor[1]
   b. 85–120 bpm with good variability during the second stage of labor
2. Congenital complete heart block
   a. Associated with high incidence of structural heart lesions[2]
   b. Associated with maternal connective tissue disease (esp SLE) present or future (in 33%–50%)[3–4]
   c. Maternal viral infection
   d. Maternal hypothermia
3. β-adrenergic blocking drugs (propranolol)
4. Central nervous system anomalies
5. Prolonged deceleration
6. Fetal death (with transmitted maternal signal)

Selected references:

1. Young BK, et al: Fetal blood and tissue pH with moderate bradycardia, *Am J Obstet Gynecol* 1979; 135:45.
2. Shenker L: Fetal cardiac arrhythmias, *Obstet Gynecol Survey* 1979; 34:561.
3. Chamedes L, et al: Association of maternal SLE with congenital complete heart block, *N Engl J Med* 1977; 297:1204.
4. McCue CM, et al: Congenital heart block in newborns of mothers with connective tissue disease. *Circulation* 1977; 56:82.

*From Main DM, Main EK: *Obstetrics and Gynecology. A Pocket Reference.* St Louis, Mosby–Year Book, 1984. Used by permission.

TABLE K–5.
Clinical Conditions Associated With the Sudden Onset of Prolonged Fetal Decelerations*

1. Severe fetal hypoxia
2. Uterine hyperstimulation (spontaneous or oxytocin induced)
3. Prolapsed umbilical cord
4. Regional anesthetic—paracervical or epidural (intravascular toxic effects or local vasoconstriction)
5. Supine hypotension
6. Vaginal examination
7. Application of an internal fetal scalp electrode or fetal scalp blood sampling
8. Maternal convulsion
9. Maternal respiratory arrest (high spinal, IV narcotic)
10. Prolonged umbilical cord compression associated with rapid descent of the fetus during expulsion

*From Main DM, Main EK: *Obstetrics and Gynecology. A Pocket Reference.* St Louis, Mosby–Year Book, 1984. Used by permission.

TABLE K–6.

Causes of Fetal Tachycardia*

1. Fetal hypoxia
2. Amnionitis or fetal infection
3. Maternal fever
4. Parasympatholytic drugs
   a. Atropine
   b. Sedative drugs
   c. Vistaril/Atarax
   d. Phenothiazines
5. Beta-Sympathomimetic drugs
   a. Terbutaline
   b. Ritodrine
6. Fetal anemia
7. Fetal heart failure
8. Fetal cardiac tachyarrhythmia
9. Maternal hyperthyroidism

*From Main DM, Main EK: *Obstetrics and Gynecology. A Pocket Reference.* St Louis, Mosby–Year Book, 1984. Used by permission.

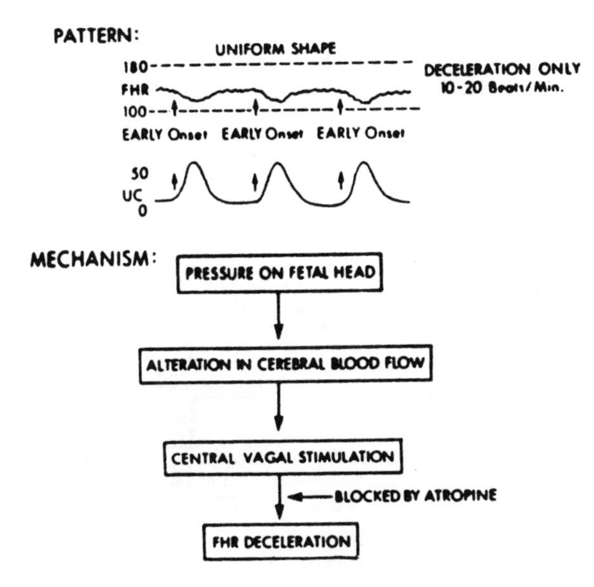

FIG K–1.

Pattern and mechanism of early decelerations. Early decelerations generally occur at 4 to 7 cm of cervical dilation. They can be reproduced by pressing a doughnut pessary with an internal diameter of 4 to 6 cm over the neonatal head, causing compression of the anterior fontanelle. This pattern is not associated with fetal hypoxia, acidosis, or low Apgar scores. (Modified from Freeman RK, Garite TJ: *Fetal Heart Rate Monitoring*. Baltimore, Williams & Wilkins, 1981, p 13; and Hon EH: *Atlas of Fetal Heart Rate Patterns*. New Haven, Harty Press, 1968, p 51. As published in Main DM, Main EK: *Obstetrics and Gynecology. A Pocket Reference*. St Louis, Mosby–Year Book, 1984. Used by permission.)

PATTERN:

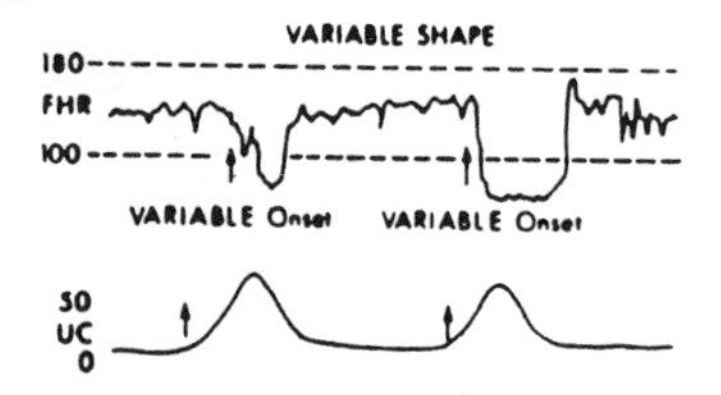

MECHANISM:

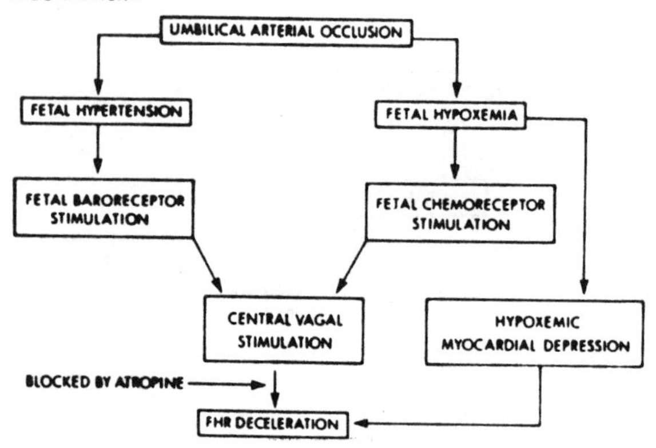

FIG K–2.

Pattern and mechanism of variable decelerations. Variable decelerations are variable in duration, intensity, and timing relative to contractions. Characteristically, they are abrupt in onset and return to baseline. The degree of fetal compromise will vary directly with the duration and degree of cord compression. If compression is prolonged and repetitive, fetal hypoxia and acidosis may occur. Associated loss of variability and tachycardia suggest fetal compromise. (Modified from Freeman RK, Garite TJ: *Fetal Heart Rate Monitoring*. Baltimore, Williams & Wilkins, 1981, p 15; and Hon EH: *Atlas of Fetal Heart Rate Patterns*. New Haven, Harty Press, 1968, p 51. As published in Main DM, Main EK: *Obstetrics and Gynecology. A Pocket Reference*. St Louis, Mosby–Year Book, 1984. Used by permission.)

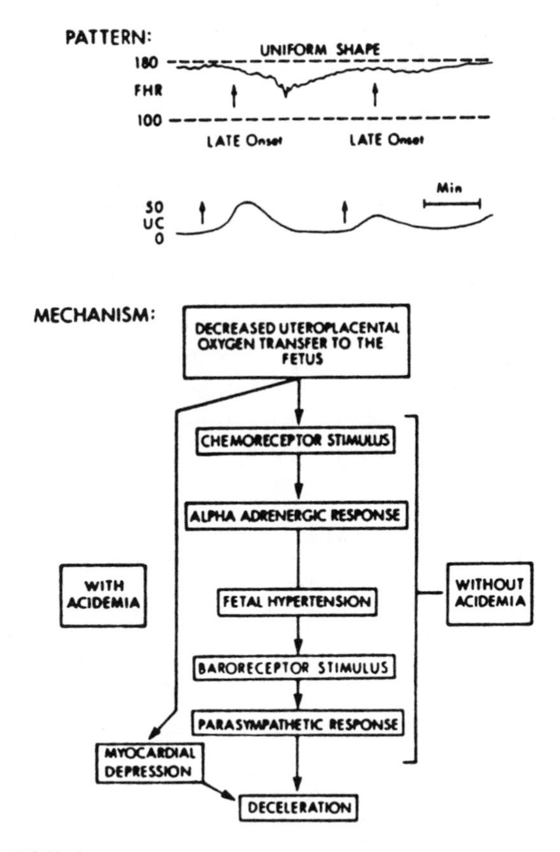

FIG K–3.

Pattern and mechanism of late decelerations. (Modified from Freeman RK, Garite TJ: *Fetal Heart Rate Monitoring*. Baltimore, Williams & Wilkins, 1981, p 15; and Hon EH: *Atlas of Fetal Heart Rate Patterns*. New Haven, Harty Press, 1968, p 51. As published in Main DM, Main EK: *Obstetrics and Gynecology. A Pocket Reference*. St Louis, Mosby–Year Book, 1984. Used by permission.)

APPENDIX L: ANTEPARTUM FETAL SURVEILLANCE

I. Background

A. Seventy percent of fetal deaths occur before the onset of labor. Antepartum surveillance is designed to identify those fetuses at risk of intrauterine compromise and death at a time when intervention could improve fetal outcome.

1. Causes of stillbirth include:
   a. Chronic uteroplacental insufficiency (UPI) 60%–70%
   b. Congenital anomalies 20%–25%
   c. Acute UPI (abruptio placentae, placenta previa, or infection) 5%–10%
   d. Unexplained 5%–10%
2. Acute events that occur randomly or suddenly may not be identifiable by antepartum testing. These events include:
   a. Cord accidents
   b. Abruptio placentae
   c. Hydrops fetalis
   d. Intrauterine infection

B. Candidates for Testing

1. It is not practical to monitor all patients. Patients at high risk for UPI are appropriate candidates for antepartum testing. Those with the most serious and unpredictable conditions require testing soon after fetal viability. When a disorder that predisposes to UPI is diagnosed during pregnancy (i.e. preeclampsia), begin testing at the time of diagnosis.
   a. Conditions that indicate the need for testing at a specific time:

1) Diabetes, classes A_2–R	32–33 wk
2) Diabetes class A, complicated by hypertension	32–34 wk
3) Chronic hypertension	32–34 wk
4) Autoimmune disease	32–34 wk
5) Maternal cardiac disease	32–34 wk
6) Hemoglobinopathy	32–34 wk
7) Maternal renal disease	32–34 wk
8) Diabetes class A, uncomplicated	40 wk
9) Postdate pregnancy	42 wk

b. Conditions that indicate the need for testing upon diagnosis:
   1) Preeclampsia
   2) Suspected intrauterine growth retardation
   3) Discordant twins

c. Conditions that may indicate a need for testing, depending on the clinical setting:
   1) Decreased fetal movement
   2) Maternal age ≥35 years
   3) Rh isoimmunization
   4) Maternal hyperthyroidism

II. Surveillance Techniques

A. Fetal Movement Counts

1. Women, with term gestations, who are trained in the manner of detecting fetal movement are able to detect 85% of gross fetal movement. This mode of testing is a particularly useful surveillance tool for all patients, including those at low risk.
2. A common method of determining fetal movement is to instruct the patient to:
   a. Lie down on her left side after a meal
   b. Count the number of fetal movements that occur
   c. If less than three movements per hour for 2 consecutive hours, inform the physician

B. Nonstress Test (NST)

1. The NST monitors the fetal heart rate (FHR) in the absence of regular uterine activity. The presence of FHR accelerations is considered reassuring. The FHR is interpreted according to the level of FHR reactivity:
   a. **Reactive** identifies the fetus with:
      1) 2 FHR accelerations of 15 seconds' duration in a 20-minute period, **and**
      2) The peak amplitude of accelerations are 15 beats/min above the baseline.
   b. **Nonreactive** is the lack of either (1) or (2) (under reactive).
2. Reactivity is decreased in the presence of fetal sleep or inactivity and in gestations less than 30 weeks. Sound stimulation with an artificial larynx may arouse a resting fetus.
3. The testing interval is every 3 or 4 days.

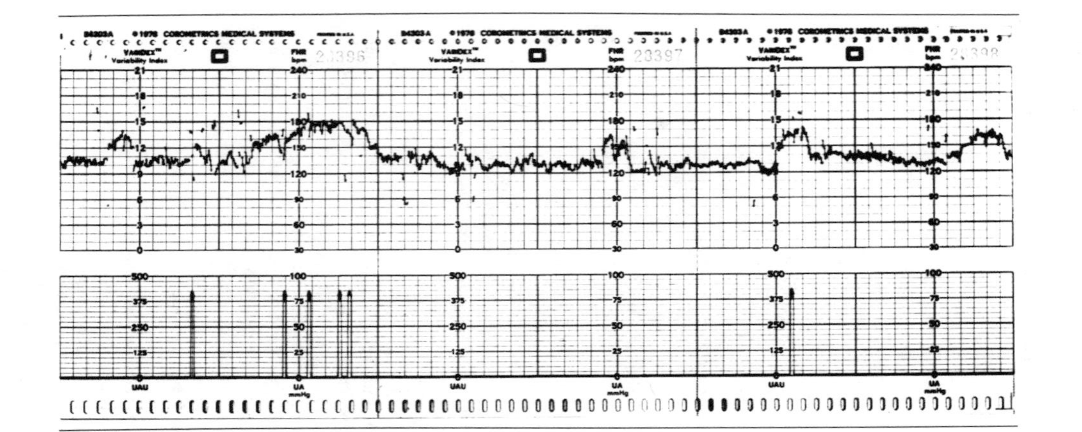

FIG L–1.

Reactive NST. Accelerations of the fetal heart that are greater than 15 beats/min and last longer than 15 seconds can be identified. When the patient appreciates a fetal movement, she presses an event marker on the monitor, creating the arrows on the lower portion of the tracing. (From Gabbe SG, Niebyl JR, Simpson JL: *Obstetrics: Normal and Problem Pregnancies*. New York, Churchill Livingstone, 1986. Used by permission.)

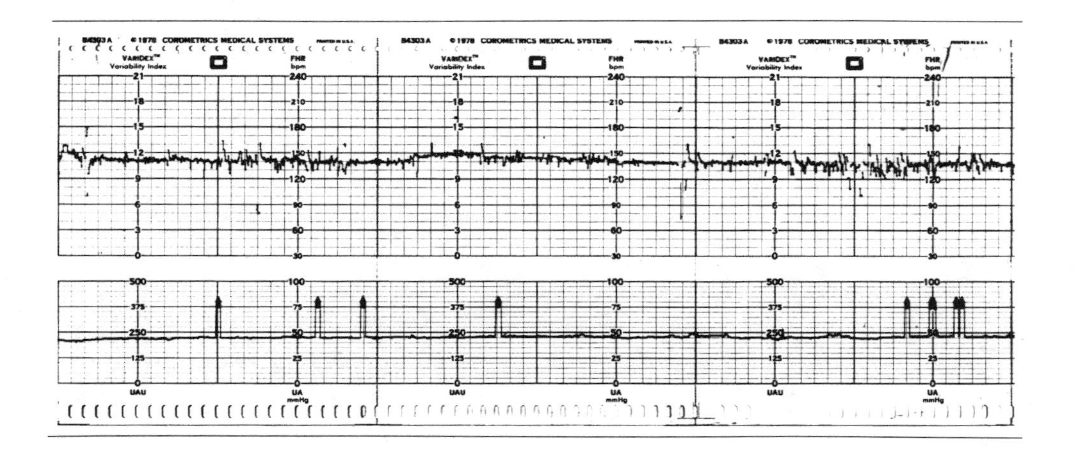

FIG L–2.
Nonreactive NST. No accelerations of the fetal heart rate are observed. The patient has perceived fetal activity as indicated by the arrows in the lower portion of the tracing. (From Gabbe SG, Niebyl JR, Simpson JL: *Obstetrics: Normal and Problem Pregnancies*. New York, Churchill Livingstone, 1986. Used by permission.)

4. The false-negative rate is 1.9–8.6/1,000 (fetal deaths within 3 or 4 days after a reactive test).

C. Contraction Stress Test (CST)

1. The CST evaluates fetal oxygen reserves. In the presence of a uterine contraction >25 mm Hg, blood is restricted in its flow through the uterus. Fetuses with adequate oxygen reserves tolerate the stress of a uterine contraction, but those with diminished reserves demonstrate a fall in heart rate.
2. A CST may be performed weekly if the results are reactive negative, except in diabetic patients in whom a mid week NST is recommended.
3. An absolute contraindication to a CST is a previous classical cesarean section or other uterine surgery where the endometrial cavity was entered. The exception is a low transverse cesarean section.

TABLE L–1.

Interpretation of the Contraction Stress Test*

Interpretation	Description	Incidence (%)
Negative	No late decelerations appearing anywhere on the tracing with adequate uterine contractions (3 in 10 minutes)	80
Positive	Late decelerations that are consistent and persistent, present with the majority (greater than 50 percent) of contractions without excessive uterine activity; if persistent late decelerations are seen before the frequency of contractions is adequate, the test is interpreted as positive	3–5
Suspicious	Inconsistent late decelerations	5
Hyperstimulation	Uterine contractions closer than every 2 minutes or lasting greater than 90 seconds, or 5 uterine contractions in 10 minutes; if no late decelerations seen, test interpreted as negative	5
Unsatisfactory	Quality of the tracing inadequate for interpretation, or adequate uterine activity cannot be achieved	5

*From Gabbe SG, Niebyl JR, Simpson JL: *Obstetrics: Normal and Problem Pregnancies.* New York, Churchill Livingstone, 1986. Used by permission.

TABLE L–2.
Testing Scheme: CST

CST			
Negative	Equivocal	Positive Reactive	Nonreactive
Repeat in 1 wk	Repeat in 1 day	If term or amniocentesis demonstrates pulmonary maturity, deliver If fetus is immature, repeat the CST	Consider delivery

D. Biophysical Profile (BPP)

1. In a BPP, fetal biophysical parameters are studied ultrasonically, and five independent variables that correlate with fetal well being are investigated.
2. The technique of the BPP scoring is detailed in Table L–3, suggested management based on result of the BPP in Table L–4, and testing scheme.
3. Studies have demonstrated that
   a. Fetuses with low scores are frequently acidotic.
   b. Higher scores (8 and 10) usually indicate that the fetus is healthy. The false-negative rate is 1–2/1,000 (these fetuses die within 7 days of a reassuring test).
   c. In patients with premature rupture of membranes, absent fetal breathing is predictive of fetal infection.
   d. Equivocal tests are uncommon.
   e. No contraindications exist to the test.
4. The BPP testing interval is 7 days, except in patients with diabetes, significant intrauterine growth retardation, or a postdates fetus where testing is recommended every 3 to 4 days.

E. Modified BPP

1. The modified BPP includes both a NST and calculation of the amniotic fluid volume (AFV) (Fig L–3). Clinical results and failure rates are similar to those obtained with a full BPP. Estimations of the AFV correlate well with the actual fluid volume and fetal outcome. Perinatal mortality rates have been demonstrated to correlate well with the amniotic fluid index (AFI) (Table L–5).

TABLE L–3.
Technique of Biophysical Profile Scoring*

Biophysical Variable	Normal (Score = 2)	Abnormal (Score = 0)
Fetal breathing movements	At least one episode of at least 30 seconds duration in 30 minutes observation	Absent or no episode of ≥30 seconds duration in 30 minutes
Gross body movement	At least three discrete body/limb movements in 30 minutes (episodes of active continuous movement considered a single movement)	Up to two episodes of body/limb movements in 30 minutes
Fetal tone	At least one episode of active extension with return to flexion of fetal limb(s) or trunk; opening and closing of hand considered normal tone	Either slow extension with return to partial flexion or movement of limb in full extension or absent fetal movement
Reactive fetal heart rate	At least two episodes of acceleration of ≥15 bpm and at least 15 seconds duration associated with fetal movement in 30 minutes	Fewer than two accelerations or acceleration <15 bpm in 30 minutes
Qualitative amniotic fluid volume	At least one pocket of amniotic fluid measuring at least 1 cm in two perpendicular planes	Either no amniotic fluid pockets or a pocket <1 cm in two perpendicular planes

*Adapted from Manning F, Baskett T, Morrison I, et al: *Am J Obstet Gynecol* 1981; 140:289. As published in Gabbe SG, Niebyl JR, Simpson JL: *Obstetrics: Normal and Problem Pregnancies.* New York, Churchill Livingstone, 1986. Used by permission.

TABLE L–4.

Management Based on the Biophysical Profile*

Score	Interpretation	Management
10	Normal infant; low risk of chronic asphyxia	Repeat testing at weekly intervals; repeat twice weekly in diabetics and patients at ≥42 weeks' gestation.
8	Normal infant; low risk of chronic asphyxia	Repeat testing at weekly intervals; repeat testing twice weekly in diabetics and patients at ≥42 weeks' gestation; oligohydramnios is an indication for delivery.
6	Suspect chronic asphyxia	Repeat testing within 24 hours; deliver if oligohydramnios is present.
4	Suspect chronic asphyxia	If ≥36 weeks' gestation and conditions are favorable, deliver; if at <36 weeks and L/S <2.0, repeat test same day; if repeat score ≤4, deliver.
0–2	Strongly suspect chronic asphyxia	Extend testing time to 120 minutes; if persistent score ≤4, deliver, regardless of gestational age.

*Adapted from Manning F, Baskett T, Morrison I, et al: *Am J Obstet Gynecol* 1981; 140:289. As published in Gabbe SG, Niebyl JR, Simpson JL: *Obstetrics: Normal and Problem Pregnancies.* New York, Churchill Livingstone, 1986. Used by permission.

MODIFIED BIOPHYSICAL PROFILE

Nonstress Test (NST) Twice per Week
and
Amniotic Fluid Index (AFI) Once per Week

↓

If Nonreactive NST or AFI < 5 cm

↓

Backup Test
Contraction Stress Test (CST)
or
Biophysical Profile (BPP)

↓

Manage as With BPP or CST

FIG L–3.
Modified BPP decision tree.

TABLE L–5.
Relationship of Amniotic Fluid Levels to Perinatal Mortality Rates

Amniotic Fluid Index*	Perinatal Mortality Rate
Normal (8–24 cm)	1.97/1,000
Marginal (5–8 cm)	37.74/1,000
Decreased (<5 cm)	109.4/1,000

*The Amniotic Fluid Index (AFI) is the measurement, in centimeters, of the deepest fluid pockets found in all four quadrants of the uterus, as demonstrated on ultrasound with the transducer perpendicular to the floor.

TABLE L–6.

Summary of Antepartum Fetal Surveillance Modalities

Test	Patient Indications	Testing Interval	Equipment Required	Expertise Required	Equivocal Results	False-Negative Rate	Cost
FMC	Low risk	Daily	None	Minimal	—	—	None
NST	High risk	3–4 days	1. FHR monitor	Intermed.	Frequent	1.9–8.6/1,000	Modest
CST	High risk	Weekly	1. FHR monitor 2. Possible IV infusion	Intermed.	Frequent	0–2.2/1,000	Modest
BPP	High risk	Weekly	1. FHR monitor 2. Ultrasound	Advanced	Uncommon	1–2/1,000	Expensive
Mod BPP	High risk	3–4 days	1. FHR monitor 2. Ultrasound	Advanced	Uncommon	1–2/1,000	Expensive

FMC = fetal movement count; NST = nonstress test; CST = contraction stress test; BPP = biophysical profile; Mod BPP = modified biophysical profile.

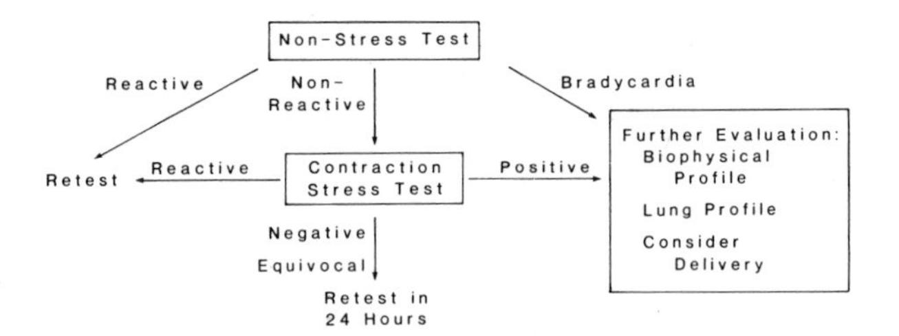

FIG L–4.
Branched testing scheme with use of the NST, CST, and BPP. Delivery is considered when the NST result is nonreactive and the CST results are positive. Delivery is also considered when a bradycardia is observed during the NST. The fetal BPP may be used to decrease the incidence of unnecessary premature intervention. (From Gabbe SG, Niebyl JR, Simpson JL: *Obstetrics: Normal and Problem Pregnancies*. New York, Churchill Livingstone, 1986. Used by permission.)

2. All modalities for calculating the AFV include measuring the largest pocket of fluid while the ultrasound transducer is held perpendicular to the floor. The AFI (Rutherford and Phelan) is the sum of the depths (in centimeters) of the amniotic fluid in the four abdominal quadrants, divided at the umbilicus (from 30 weeks' gestation onward). A rough guide for fluid volume determination is:

a. AFI <5 cm per quadrant = oligohydramnios.
b. AFI 5–8 cm per quadrant = borderline oligohydramnios.
c. AFI 8–25 cm = normal.
d. AFI >25 cm per quadrant = polyhydramnios.

F. A summary of antepartum fetal surveillance modalities is shown in Table L–6, and a branched scheme for using the NST, CST, and modified BPP in Fig L–4.

APPENDIX M: FETAL LUNG MATURITY: GLUCOCORTICOIDS FOR ACCELERATED FETAL LUNG MATURATION

I. Fetal Lung Maturity

A. Fetal lung maturity may be determined by analyzing a specimen of amniotic fluid (usually obtained by amniocentesis).
B. The methods of assessing fetal lung maturity are detailed in Tables M–1 and M–2.
C. Modifiers of pulmonary maturity tests are detailed in Table M–3.
D. The relationship of phospholipid production, phosphatidylinositol, and phosphatidylglycerol in amniotic fluid, and the lecithin/sphingomyelin (L/S) ratio, are detailed in Figs M–1, M–2, and M–3. When determining the lung maturity in infants of diabetic mothers, an L/S ratio higher than that of nondiabetic patients is required. The absolute value is dependent on the institution in which the study is performed.
E. The foam stability, or "shake" test, is detailed in Figs M–4 and M–5.

II. Glucocorticoids for Accelerated Fetal Lung Maturation

A. Antenatal steroids have been demonstrated to reduce the incidence of respiratory distress syndrome and neonatal deaths in infants delivered between 28 and 34 weeks' gestation.
B. A comparison of corticosteroids is shown in Table M–4. The primary glucocorticoids used are:
   1. **Betamethasone,** 12 mg IM every 24 hours times two total doses
   2. **Dexamethasone,** 5 mg IM every 12 hours times four total doses
C. Fetal and Neonatal Effects
   1. Delivery must occur between 2 and 7 days after administration of the first dose of steroid for the beneficial effect to be present.
   2. A significant reduction in respiratory distress syndrome is noted in female infants, while white male infants receive no apparent benefit.
   3. No increase in the incidence of neonatal infections has been noted. A slight increase in the infection rate might be

TABLE M–1.
Assessment of Fetal Lung Maturity: Principle and Levels of Maturity*

Test	Principle	Mature Level
L/S ratio	Quantity of surfactant lecithin compared with sphingomyelin	≥2.0 (method dependent)
Lung profile	Includes determination of L/S ratio, percentage precipitable lecithin, PG and PI	L/S ratio ≥2.0; >50% acetone precipitable lecithin, 15–20% PI, 2–10% PG
Amniostat-FLM†	Immunologic test with agglutination in presence of PG	Test positive with PG ≥ 2 μg/mL amniotic fluid
Disaturated phosphatidylcholine (DSPC)	Direct measure of primary phospholipid in surfactant	≥500 μg/dL
Microviscosimeter†	Fluorescence depolarization used to determine phospholipid membrane content	$P < 0.310–0.336$
Shake test†	Generation of stable foam by pulmonary surfactant in presence of ethanol	Complete ring of bubbles 15 minutes after shaking at 1:2 dilution
Lumadex-FSI†	Modification of manual foam stability index; stable foam in presence of increasing concentration of ethanol	≥47
Optical density†	Evaluates turbidity changes dependent on total phospholipid concentration	At 650 nm, ≥0.15

*Adapted from Gabbe S: *J Reprod Med* 1979; 23:277. As published in Gabbe SG, Niebyl JR, Simpson JL: *Obstetrics: Normal and Problem Pregnancies*. New York, Churchill Livingstone, 1986. Used by permission.
†Denotes screening test.
L/S = Lecithin/sphingomyelin; PG = phosphatidylglycerol; PI = phosphatidylinositol.

TABLE M–2.

Assessment of Fetal Lung Maturity: Testing Modality Advantages and Disadvantages*

Test	Advantages	Disadvantages
L/S ratio	Few falsely mature values: not altered by changes in amniotic fluid volume	Many falsely immature values, long turnaround time, special laboratory equipment required
Lung profile	Reduces falsely immature L/S ratios: PG not altered by blood, meconium	Requires more time and equipment than L/S ratio
Amniostat-FLM†	Rapid, few falsely mature tests: can be used with contaminated specimens	Many falsely immature results
Disaturated phosphatidylcholine (DSPC)	Few falsely mature tests: may reduce falsely immature tests	May be altered by changes in amniotic fluid volume
Microviscosimeter†	Few falsely mature tests; fast, easily performed	Requires expensive equipment
Shake test†	Few falsely mature tests; fast, easily performed	Concentration of reagents critical; many falsely immature results
Lumadex-FSI†	Few falsely mature tests; fast, easily performed	Concentration of reagents critical; some falsely immature results
Optical density at 650 nm†	Few falsely mature tests; fast, easily performed	Many falsely immature results; need clear amniotic fluid

*Adapted from Gabbe S: *J Reprod Med* 1979; 23:277. As published in Gabbe SG, Niebyl JR, Simpson JL: *Obstetrics: Normal and Problem Pregnancies.* New York, Churchill Livingstone, 1986. Used by permission.

†Denotes screening test.

LS = lecithin/sphingomyelin; PG = phosphatidylglycerol.

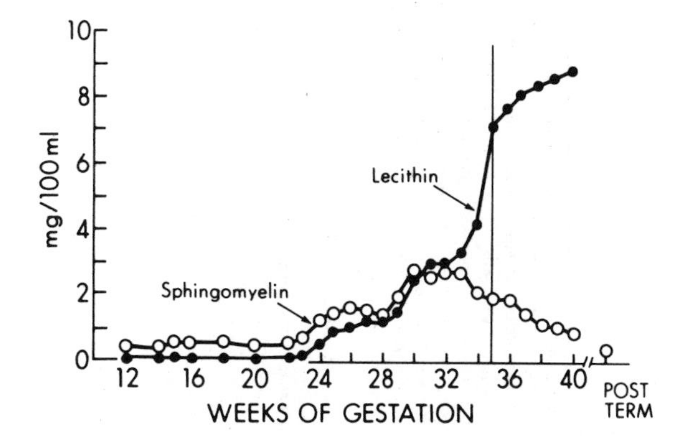

FIG M–1.

Phospholipid production vs gestational age in normal pregnancies. Changes in mean concentrations of lecithin and sphingomyelin in amniotic fluid in normal pregnancy. (From Gluck L, Kulovich MV: *Am J Obstet Gynecol* 1973; 115:539. Used by permission.)

TABLE M–3.

Modifiers of Pulmonary Maturity Tests* †

Test	Blood	Meconium	Temperature	Collection Location
L/S	Inconsistent effect appears to raise immature L/S & lower mature L/S. L/S ratio of serum is 1.31–1.46.[1]	Inconsistent effect reported to increase L/S by 0.1–0.5, effect more pronounced in term infants.[10]	Room temperature storage × 24 hrs may decrease L/S.[2] However another study[3] suggests L/S stable at 22 C (room temp) × 72 hr, 4 C × 72 hr and −40 C for 1 yr.	Vaginal collection of free-flowing amniotic fluid is reliable.[4] Amniocentesis near fetal mouth may increase L/S relative to collection far from fetal mouth.[5]
PG	Reliable even in face of bloody fluid.[6]		Tendency to decrease PG at room temp, but decrease not significant. Stable at 4 C × 48 hr and at −20 C × 1 yr.[3]	Vaginal samples clinically reliable.[7]
Shake	May produce falsely mature results.[8]	May produce falsely mature results.[8]	Reliable at 20 to 30 C range. Lower temps increase "maturity" and higher temps decrease "maturity" (bubble stability).[8]	
Saturated Phosphotidylcholine	Reliable.[9]	Reliable.[9]		

Selected references:

1. Buhi WC, Spellacy WN: Effects of blood or meconium on the determination of the amniotic fluid lecithin/sphingomyelin ratio, *Am J Obstet Gynecol* 1975; 121:321.
2. Kulkarni BD, et al.: Determination of lecithin-sphingomyelin ratio in amniotic fluid, *Obstet Gynecol* 1972; 40:173.
3. Schwartz DB, et al.: The stability of phospholipids in amniotic fluid, *Am J Obstet Gynecol* 1981; 141:294.
4. Srerra AJ, et al: The effect of cervical/vaginal secretions on measurements of lecithin/sphingomyelin ratio and optical density at 650 nm, *Am J Obstet Gynecol* 1981; 139:214.
5. Worthington D, Smith BT: The site of amniocentesis and the lecithin-sphingomyelin ratio, *Obstet Gynecol* 1978; 52:552.
6. Strassner HT, Jr, et al: Effect of blood in amniotic fluid on the detection of phosphatidylglycerol. *Am J Obstet Gynecol* 1980; 138:697.
7. Stedman CM, et al: Management of preterm premature rupture of membranes: Assessing amniotic fluid in the vagina for phosphatidylglycerol. *Am J Obstet Gynecol* 1981; 140:34.
8. Keniston RC, Noland GL, Pernoll ML: The effect of blood, meconium and temperature on the rapid surfactant test, *Obstet Gynecol* 1976; 48:442.
9. Torday J, Carson L, Lawson EE: Saturated phosphatidylcholine in amniotic fluid and prediction of respiratory distress syndrome. *N Engl J Med* 1979; 301:1013.
10. Tabsh KMA, Brinkman CR, Bashore R: Effect of meconium contamination on amniotic fluid lecithin: Sphingomyelin ratio, *Obstet Gynecol* 1981; 58:605.

*From Main DM, Main EK: *Obstetrics and Gynecology. A Pocket Reference.* St Louis, Mosby–Year Book, 1984. Used by permission.
†LS = lecithin/sphingomyelin; PG = phosphatidylglycerol.

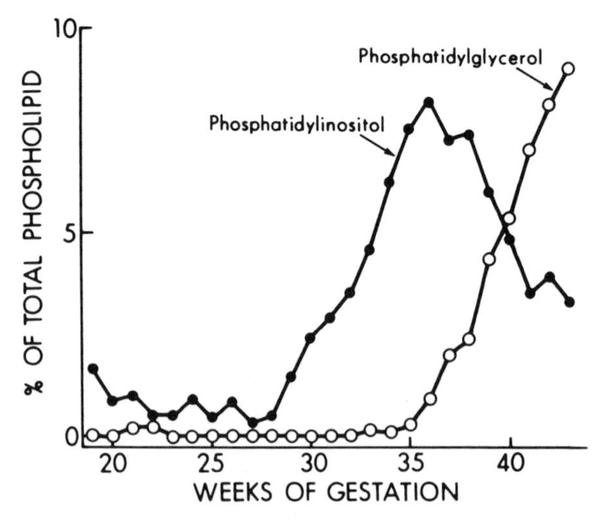

FIG M–2.
The content of phosphatidylinositol and phosphatidylglycerol in amniotic fluid during normal gestation. The phospholipids were quantified by measuring the phosphorus (P) content and expressed as percentages of total lipid phosphorus. Mean ± standard deviations of three to five samples are shown for each point. Phosphatidylglycerol appears to be important as a "stabilizer" for other lecithins, especially in the face of acidosis and maternal diabetes. Phosphatidylinositol's only clinical importance is to mark a sample as "not-fully-mature." (From Hallman M, et al: *Am J Obstet Gynecol* 1976; 125:613. Used by permission.)

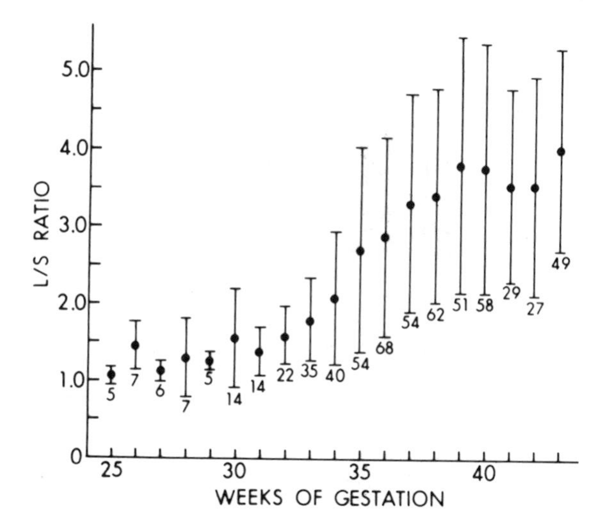

FIG M–3.

L/S vs gestational age in 607 samples of amniotic fluid from 425 patients. Gestational age is given by the best antepartum estimate. One standard deviation is shown. The numbers immediately below the standard deviation bars indicate the number of amniotic fluid samples used for the computation at each corresponding week of gestation. These results are quite comparable to Figure M–1. Note that in both graphs the mean age of a mature L/S ratio (2.0) is 34 to 35 weeks. (From Donald IR, et al: *Am J Obstet Gynecol* 1973; 115:547. Used by permission.)

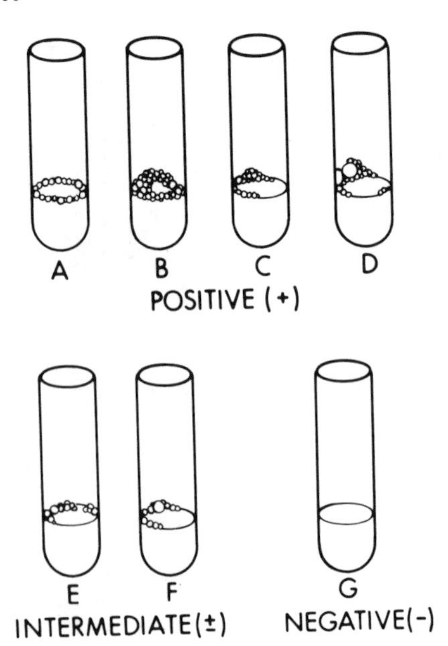

FIG M–4.
Foam stability or "shake" test. (From Main DM, Main EK: *Obstetrics and Gynecology. A Pocket Reference*. St Louis, Mosby–Year Book, 1984. Used by permission.)

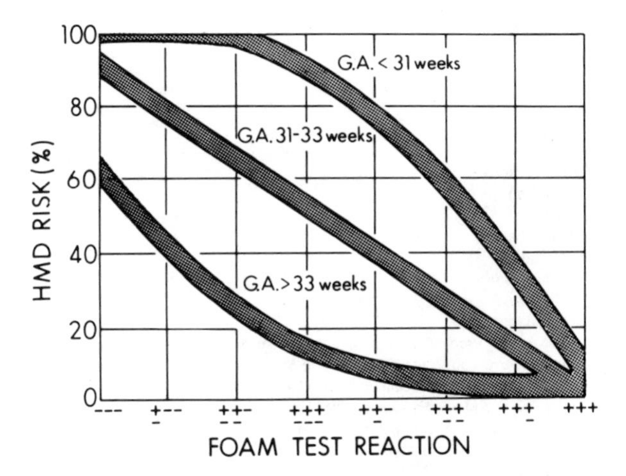

FIG M–5.
Risk of developing RDS based on "shake" test and gestational age. This graph allows for antenatal prediction of risk for hyaline membrane disease (HMD) from amniotic fluid foam test reaction at a given gestational age *(GA)*. Foam test reaction is on the longitudinal axis and risk of HMD on the vertical axis. The risk is predicted from the shaded band appropriate for GA. The width of each band approximates the error of the estimate. For example, with foam test reaction of ± ± ± the risk of HMD is approximately 15% if the GA is 33 weeks, 55% if the GA is 31 to 33 weeks, and approximately 90% if it is 31 weeks. This figure is based on experience with 410 infants, 64 of whom developed hyaline membrane disease, and all of whom had the "shake" test performed within 24 hours of delivery. (From Schleuter MA, et al: *Am J Obstet Gynecol* 1979; 134:761. Used by permission.)

TABLE M–4.

Comparison of Corticosteroids*

Compounds	Equivalent Dose†	Anti-Inflammatory Potency‡	Relative Sodium Retaining Potency‡	Maternal-Fetal Gradient[1]
Hydrocortisone (Cortisol)	20 mg	1.0	1.0	5.8:1
Prednisone	5 mg	4.0	0.8	10:1
Dexamethasone (Decadron)	0.75 mg	25.0	0	
Betamethasone (Celestone)	0.75 mg	25.0	0	3:1

Selected references:

1. Ballard PC: Prenatal glucocorticoid treatment: Maternal and infant cord blood cortisol levels, in Moore TC (ed): *Lung Maturation and Prevention of Hyaline Membrane Disease.* Columbus, Ross Laboratories, 1976, p 89.
2. Haynes RC, Murad F: Adrenocorticotropic hormone; Adrenocortical steroids and their synthetic analogs; inhibitors of adrenocortical steroid biosynthesis, in Gilman AG, Goodman LS, Gilman A (eds): *The Pharmacological Basis of Therapeutics,* ed 6, New York, MacMillan, 1980, p 1482.

*From Main DM, Main EK: *Obstetrics and Gynecology. A Pocket Reference.* St Louis, Mosby–Year Book, 1984. Used by permission.

†Equivalent to 5 mg prednisone, usual adrenal replacement dose. (Note that 12 mg betamethasone or dexamethasone equals 80 mg of prednisone.)[2]

‡Compared to hydrocortisone.[2]

TABLE M–5.

Effect of Short Course Steroid Administration on Maternal WBC and Differential* †

	WBC/mm^3	
	Mean	+2SD
Pretreatment	10,576	15,854
Posttreatment	13,185	18,821
% Mean change	↑ 25%	

*From Wong YC, Taeusch HW: *Pediatr Res* 1978; 12:501. As published in Main DM, Main EK: *Obstetrics and Gynecology. A Pocket Reference.* St Louis, Mosby–Year Book, 1984. Used by permission.

†The mean increase in WBC with steroid therapy was accompanied by a 40% mean increase in neutrophils and a 35% mean decrease in lymphocytes. This data is based on serial values from 20 patients treated with dexamethasone 4 mg IM q 8 hr × 6 doses and 20 patients treated with saline IM q 8 hr × 6 doses who served as double blind controls.

present if premature rupture of membranes is present when the steroids are administered.

4. A reduction in intraventricular hemorrhage and the patent ductus arteriosus rate has been noted.
5. Follow-up of the children treated in utero demonstrates no physical, cognitive, or psychologic impairment.

D. Maternal Effects

1. The maternal infection rate is not increased when glucocorticoids are used for fetal lung maturation, except possibly when premature rupture of membranes is present before steroid administration (Table M–5).
2. Glucose intolerance may develop temporarily.

BIBLIOGRAPHY

Collaborative Group on Antenatal Steroid Therapy: Effect of antenatal dexamethasone administration on the prevention of respiratory distress syndrome. *Am J Obstet Gynecol* 1981; 141:276.

Farrell EE, Silver RK, Kimberlin LV, et al: Impact of antenatal dexamethasone administration on respiratory distress syndrome in surfactant-treated infants. *Am J Obstet Gynecol* 1989; 161:628–633.

Gabbe SG, Niebyl JR, Simpson JL. *Obstetrics: Normal and Problem Pregnancies*. New York, Churchill Livingstone, 1986.

Garite TJ, Freeman RK, Linzey EM, et al: Prospective randomized study of corticosteroids in the management of premature rupture of the membranes and the premature gestation. *Am J Obstet Gynecol* 1981; 141:508.

Loggins GC, Howie RN: A controlled trial of antepartum glucocorticoid treatment for prevention of the respiratory distress syndrome in premature infants. *Pediatrics* 1972; 50:515.

APPENDIX N: FETAL LUNG MATURITY: ASSESSMENT BEFORE REPEAT CESAREAN DELIVERY*

The assessment of fetal maturity is an important in determining the timing of a repeat cesarean delivery. For patients being considered for elective repeat cesarean deliveries, if one of the following criteria is met, fetal maturity may be assumed and amniocentesis need not be performed:

1. Fetal heart tones have been documented for 20 weeks by nonelectronic fetoscope or for 30 weeks by Doppler.
2. It has been 36 weeks since a positive serum or urine human chorionic gonadotropin pregnancy test was performed by a reliable laboratory.
3. An ultrasound measurement of the crown-rump length, obtained at 6–11 weeks, supports a gestational age of ≥ 39 weeks.
4. An ultrasound, obtained at 12–20 weeks, confirms the gestational age of ≥ 39 weeks determined by clinical history and physical examination.

These criteria are not intended to preclude the use of menstrual dating. If any one of the above criteria confirms gestational age assessment on the basis of menstrual dates in a patient with normal menstrual cycles and no immediately antecedent use of oral contraceptives, it is appropriate to schedule delivery at ≥ 39 weeks by the menstrual dates. Ultrasound may be considered confirmatory of menstrual dates if there is gestational age agreement within 1 week by crown-rump measurement obtained at 6–11 weeks or within 10 days by the average of multiple measurements obtained at 12–20 weeks.†

Awaiting the onset of spontaneous labor is another option.

*Committee Opinion Number 98, September, 1991. Committee on Obstetrics: Maternal and Fetal Medicine. Copyright September, 1991, The American College of Obstetrics and Gynecologists, Washington, DC.

†American College of Obstetritions and Gynecologists. Ultrasound in pregnancy. ACOG Technical Bulletin 116. Washington, DC, ACOG, 1988.

MEDICATION ADMINISTRATION

APPENDIX O: MEDICATIONS IN PREGNANCY: FDA GUIDELINES*

TABLE O–1.

Medications in Pregnancy: FDA's "Pregnancy Categories"

Category A: Controlled studies in women fail to demonstrate a risk to the fetus in the first trimester (and there is no evidence of a risk in later trimesters), *and* the possibility of fetal harm appears remote.

Category B: Either animal-reproduction studies have not demonstrated a fetal risk and there are no controlled studies in pregnant women, *or* animal-reproduction studies have shown an adverse effect (other than a decrease in fertility) that was not confirmed in controlled studies in women in the first trimester (and there is no evidence of a risk in later trimesters).

Category C: Either studies in animals have revealed adverse effects on the fetus (teratogenic or embryocidal effects or other) and there are no controlled studies in women, *or* studies in women and animals are not available. Drugs should be given only if the potential benefit justifies the potential risk to the fetus.

Category D: There is positive evidence of human fetal risk, but the benefits from use in pregnant women may be acceptable despite the risk (e.g., if the drug is needed in a life-threatening situation or for a serious disease for which safer drugs cannot be used or are ineffective). There will be an appropriate statement in the "warnings" section of the labeling.

Category X: Studies in animals or human beings have demonstrated fetal abnormalities or there is evidence of fetal risk based on human experience, or both, *and* the risk of the use of the drug in pregnant women clearly outweighs any possible benefit. The drug is contraindicated in women who are or may become pregnant. There will be an appropriate statement in the "contraindications" section of the labeling.

*From Main DM, Main EK: *Obstetrics and Gynecology. A Pocket Reference.* St Louis, Mosby–Year Book, 1984. Used by permission.

APPENDIX P: IMMUNIZATIONS DURING PREGNANCY*

TABLE P–1.
Immunizations During Pregnancy

I. *Active Immunization*

A vaccine must be administered at least 7–21 days *before* exposure to allow for production of antibodies. Live attenuated virus vaccines should be used with extreme caution because of the experience with rubella vaccine.

A. Live vaccines

1. *Smallpox*—As the disease has been eradicated from the world and the vaccine may have significant risks, especially to the fetus, vaccination during pregnancy is *contraindicated.*
2. *Yellow fever*—This live attenuated vaccine is apparently harmless to pregnant women and the fetus but documentation of safety is sparse. Some recommend postponing travel to yellow fever endemic areas until after the first trimester. If a woman is exposed to risk of yellow fever infection, vaccination is *not* contraindicated at any stage of pregnancy.
3. *Poliomyelitis*—Whether pregnant women are at increased risk of poliomyelitis is debated. If poliomyelitis occurs during pregnancy, there is an increased risk of abortion and probable fetal anoxic damage. Additionally, the newborn is susceptible to polio and, if infected, has a 50% mortality rate. Presently, the only candidates for vaccination are susceptible women traveling to endemic areas (tropical and semi-tropical countries). There is debate over the optimal choice of vaccine. The live attenuated (Sabin-Oral) vaccine is recommended by some and has a good safety record. Others prefer the inactivated (Salk) vaccine on theoretical grounds. Note that vaccination requires a series of doses at one- to two-month intervals.
4. *Rubella*—Rubella in early pregnancy poses a severe threat to the fetus, and the establishment of immunity for all women of child-bearing age has been a major public health goal. Unfortunately, the attenuated virus vaccines have been found to invade placental and fetal tissues producing identifiable damage. Therefore, all rubella vaccines are *contraindicated* during or the three months before pregnancy. However, in balance, there has not yet been an infant who was exposed to the vaccine in utero who has had any birth defects or other stigmata of the congenital rubella syndrome. The vaccine may be either of low teratogenicity (under 5% or may produce an "all or nothing" effect in the first trimester i.e., abortion or normal outcome). The use of normal Ig with high rubella titer for passive immunization for exposed non-immunes has not proved satisfactory.

5. *Mumps and measles*—There are no acceptable indications for the use of these vaccines during pregnancy. While there are no documented cases of fetal damage following the use of these attenuated vaccines, virus has been isolated from the placenta following mumps vaccination.
6. *Tuberculosis vaccine (BCG)*—This is the only live bacterial vaccine in present use and has a good record of safety over many years. Pregnancy does not appear to be a contraindication to vaccination, but there are few occasions when its use in pregnancy is absolutely necessary. In the United States, women with close household contacts who have pulmonary tuberculosis are treated with chemoprophylaxis. In other countries, this situation may represent a legitimate indication for vaccination.

B. Killed vaccines

1. *Cholera*—The cholera vaccine is of questionable efficacy and is no longer required for international travel. Prevention of disease spread depends principally upon hygienic measures.
2. *Influenza*—This inactivated viral vaccine rapidly becomes obsolete because of rapid antigenic shifts of the wild viruses. Therefore, only the most current vaccine should be used. While past studies have suggested an increased morbidity and mortality of pregnant women with influenza, this has not been supported by more modern, better controlled studies. Currently recommended only for medically high risk pregnant patients.
3. *Plague*—This vaccine is only recommended for those living in or traveling through areas with high incidence of plague, or for laboratory staff working with *Yersinia pestis.* Pregnant women rarely will find themselves in these situations. There are no reported adverse effects of the vaccine on pregnancy.
4. *Pneumovax*—This is a polyvalent pneumococcal capsule polysaccharide vaccine which should be given to women with significant chronic disease (especially sickle cell disease). The advantages of pneumococcal protection in these high risk groups outweighs the limited experience in pregnant populations. To date, no adverse outcomes have been reported.
5. *Rabies*—The danger of the disease is so great (essentially 100% mortality) that the presence of pregnancy does not alter indication for prophylaxis. Each case should be reviewed individually. As the vaccine is a killed virus, theoretically the risks would be quite small. In practice there is no satisfactory data on which to base counseling. The new human diploid cell vaccine has been used in a few pregnant patients without apparent adverse effect.
6. *Tetanus-diphtheria*—A combined vaccine is recommended for use if there is no primary series or no booster within the past ten years. The vaccine is safe for use in pregnancy. Risk of disease to mother or newborn is very high (60% mortality).

(Continued.)

TABLE P–1 (cont.).

7. *Typhoid*—The typhoid and para-typhoid vaccines have been used for many years and have no confirmed ill effects during pregnancy. However, controversy remains concerning their effectiveness. Currently, typhoid vaccine is recommended only for close household contacts with a typhoid carrier or for travel to an endemic area.

II. *Passive Immunization*

Antibodies to various organisms sometimes can be given to protect against the effects of infection. Purified human immunoglobulin is preferred. This class of products has been used very successfully and safely in pregnancy though experience with some of the newer products is quite limited.

1. *Normal immunoglobulin (gamma-globulin)*—This fraction has high titers of antibody against measles, rubella, and hepatitis A. Currently, its use is recommended only for prevention of hepatitis A. One dose of 500 mg will confer protection for a period of six months. Pregnant women who are traveling to areas of high incidence, and those with institutional and household contacts should receive immunization.
2. *Tetanus immunoglobulin*—This is given to pregnant women exactly as for other individuals who are at risk of infection and have not been actively immunized.
3. *Hepatitis B immunoglobulin (HBIG)*—Because of the risks for chronic carrier status for both mother and child, HBIG should be administered within 7 days of exposure (repeated in 25 days) as for any non-pregnant person. Additionally, if the mother is a chronic carrier (particularly if HB_sAg positive), the neonate should receive HBIG as soon as possible after birth. Current investigations also indicate a role for hepatitis B inactivated vaccine for a neonate in this situation.
4. *Varicella-zoster immune globulin (VZIG)*—Congenital varicella can carry a high mortality rate (5%) if the mother contracts a primary infection within 5 days of delivery. Therefore, VZIG is indicated for infants born within 5 days of maternal rash outbreak. More controversial is the use of VZIG following first or second trimester exposure of a non-immune woman to varicella. Because varicella has been linked to a low level of fetal defects and mortality, and because of the risk of pneumonia in the mother, it is not unreasonable to give VZIG in this situation. At present, however, there are no satisfactory trials demonstrating efficacy in this setting. There has been no collection of cases to fully document safety for use in pregnancy, but it is considered safe on the basis of the use of other immune globulin preparations.

Selected references:

1. ACOG Technical Bulletin #64: Immunizations during pregnancy, May 1982.
2. Amstey MS: Immunization in pregnancy, *Clin Obstet Gynecol* 1976; 19:47.
3. Center for Disease Control: Rubella vaccination during pregnancy—United States, 1971–1981, *Morbid Mortal Weekly* Rep 1982; 31:477.
4. Hart RJC: Immunization, *Clin Obstet Gynecol* 1981; 8:421.

*From Main DM, Main EK: *Obstetrics and Gynecology. A Pocket Reference.* St Louis, Mosby–Year Book, 1984. Used by permission.

APPENDIX Q: SEXUALLY TRANSMITTED DISEASE (STD) TREATMENT GUIDELINES*

Intrauterine or perinatally transmitted STD can have fatal or severely debilitating effects on the fetus. Routine prenatal care should include an assessment for STD, which in most cases includes serologic screening for syphilis and hepatitis B, testing for chlamydia, and gonorrhea culture. Prenatal screening for HIV is indicated for all patients with risk factors for HIV or with a high-risk sexual partner; some authorities recommend HIV screening of all pregnant women.

Practical management issues are discussed in the sections pertaining to specific diseases. Pregnant women and their sexual partners should be questioned about STD and counseled about possible neonatal infections. Pregnant women with primary genital herpes infection, hepatitis B, primary cytomegalovirus (CMV) infection, or Group B streptococcal infection may need to be referred to an expert for management. In the absence of lesions or other evidence of active disease, cesarean delivery and tests for herpes simplex virus (HSV) are *not* routinely indicated for pregnant women with a history of recurrent genital herpes infection. Routine HPV screening is not recommended. For a fuller discussion of these issues, as well as for infections not transmitted sexually, refer to *Guidelines for Perinatal Care*, ed 2 (1988), jointly written and published by the American Academy of Pediatrics and the American College of Obstetricians and Gynecologists.

AIDS and HIV Infection in the General STD Setting

The acquired immunodeficiency syndrome (AIDS) is a late manifestation of infection with human immunodeficiency virus (HIV). Most people infected with HIV remain asymptomatic for long periods. HIV infection is most often diagnosed by using HIV antibody tests. Detectable antibody usually develops within 3 months after infection. Confirmed positive antibody test results mean that a person is infected with HIV and is capable of transmitting the virus to others. Although negative antibody test results usually mean a person is not infected, antibody tests cannot rule out infec-

*From *Sexually Transmitted Diseases. Treatment Guidelines*. US Department of Health and Human Services, Public Health Service, Centers for Disease Control, September, 1989. Published in *MMWR* 1989; 38:S-8.

tion from a recent exposure. If antibody testing is related to a specific exposure, the test should be repeated 3 and 6 months after the exposure.

Antibody testing for HIV begins with a screening test, usually an enzyme-linked immunosorbent assay (ELISA). If the screening test results are positive, it is followed by a more specific confirmatory test, most commonly the Western blot assay. New antibody tests are being developed and licensed that are either easier to perform or more accurate. Positive results from screening tests must be confirmed before being considered definitive.

The time between infection with HIV and development of AIDS ranges from a few months to $\geq$10 years. Most people who are infected with HIV will eventually have some symptoms related to that infection. In one cohort study, AIDS developed in 48% of a group of gay men $\leq$10 years after infection, but additional AIDS cases are expected among those who have remained AIDS-free for $>$10 years.

Therapy with zidovudine (ZDV—previously known as azidothymidine) has been shown to benefit persons in the later stages of disease (AIDS or AIDS-related conditions along with a CD4 [T4] lymphocyte count less than 200/mm^3). Serious side effects, usually anemias and cytopenias, have been common during therapy with ZDV; therefore, patients taking ZDV require careful follow-up in consultation with physicians who are familiar with ZDV therapy. Clinical trials are currently evaluating ZDV therapy for persons with asymptomatic HIV infection to see if it decreases the rate of progression to AIDS. Other trials are evaluating new drugs or combinations of drugs for persons with different stages of HIV infection, including asymptomatic infections. The complete therapeutic management of HIV infection is beyond the scope of this document.

Perinatal Infections

Infants born to women with HIV infection may also be infected with HIV; this risk is estimated to be 30%–40%. The mother in such a case may be asymptomatic and her HIV infection not recognized at delivery. Infected neonates are usually asymptomatic, and currently HIV infection cannot be readily or easily diagnosed at birth. (Positive antibody test results may reflect passively transferred maternal antibodies, and the infant must be observed over time to determine if neonatal infection is present.) Infection may not become evident until the child is 12–18 months of age. All pregnant women with a history of STD should be offered HIV counseling and testing. Recognition of HIV infection in pregnancy permits health care workers to inform patients about the risks of transmission to the infant and the risks of continuing pregnancy.

Syphilis

General Principles

Serologic Tests. Dark-field examinations and direct fluorescent antibody tests on lesions or tissue are the definitive methods for diagnosing early syphilis. Presumptive diagnosis is possible by using two types of serologic tests for syphilis: (1) treponemal (e.g., fluorescent treponemal antibody absorbed [FTA-ABS], microhemagglutination assay for antibody to *Treponema pallidum* [MHATP]) and (2) nontreponemal (e.g., Venereal Disease Research Laboratory [VDRL], rapid plasma reagin [RPR]). Neither test alone is sufficient for diagnosis. Treponemal antibody test results, once positive, usually remain so for life, regardless of treatment or disease activity. Treponemal antibody titers do not correlate with disease activity and should be reported as positive or negative. Nontreponemal antibody titers do tend to correlate with disease activity, usually rising with new infection and falling after treatment. Nontreponemal antibody test results should be reported quantitatively and titered out to a final end point rather than reported as greater than an arbitrary cutoff (e.g., >1:512). With regard to changes in nontreponemal test results, a fourfold change in titers is equivalent to a two-dilution change—e.g., from 1:16 to 1:4, or from 1:8 to 1:32.

For sequential serologic tests, the same test (e.g., VDRL or RPR) should be used, and it should be run by the same laboratory. The VDRL and RPR are equally valid, but RPR titers are often slightly higher than VDRL titers and therefore are not comparable.

Neurosyphilis cannot be accurately diagnosed from any single test. Cerebrospinal fluid (CSF) tests should include cell count, protein, and VDRL (not RPR). The CSF leukocyte count is usually elevated (>5 WBC/mm^3) when neurosyphilis is present and is a sensitive measure of the efficacy of therapy. VDRL is the standard test for CSF; ***when results are positive*** it is considered ***diagnostic*** of neurosyphilis. However, results may be negative when neurosyphilis is present and cannot be used to rule out neurosyphilis. Some experts also order an FTA-ABS; this may be less specific (more false positives) but is highly sensitive. The positive predictive value of the CSF-FTA-ABS is lower, but ***when results are negative*** this test provides evidence ***against*** neurosyphilis.

Penicillin Therapy. Penicillin is the preferred drug for treating patients with syphilis. Penicillin is the only proved therapy that has been widely used for patients with neurosyphilis, congenital syphilis, or syphilis during **pregnancy. For patients with penicillin allergy, skin testing—with desensitization, if necessary**—is optimal.

Jarisch-Herxheimer Reaction. The Jarisch-Herxheimer reaction is an acute febrile reaction, often accompanied by headache, myalgia, and other symptoms, that may occur after any therapy for syphilis, and patients should be so warned. Jarisch-Herxheimer reactions are more common in patients with early syphilis. Antipyretics may be recommended, but no proven methods exist for preventing this reaction. Pregnant patients, in particular, should be warned that early labor may occur.

Persons Exposed to Syphilis (Epidemiologic Treatment). Persons sexually exposed to a patient with early syphilis should be evaluated clinically and serologically. If the exposure occurred within the previous 90 days, the person may be infected yet seronegative, and therefore should be presumptively treated. (It may be advisable to presumptively treat persons exposed more than 90 days previously if serologic test results are not immediately available and follow-up is uncertain.) Patients who have other STDs may also have been exposed to syphilis and should have a serologic test for syphilis. The dual therapy regimen currently recommended for gonorrhea (ceftriaxone and doxycycline) is probably effective against incubating syphilis. If a different, nonpenicillin antibiotic regimen is used to treat gonorrhea, the patient should have a repeat serologic test for syphilis in 3 months.

Early Syphilis. Primary and secondary syphilis and early latent syphilis of less than 1 year's duration.

Recommended regimen.—**Benzathine penicillin** G, 2.4 million units IM, in one dose.

Follow-Up.—Treatment failures can occur with any regimen. Patients should be reexamined clinically and serologically at 3 months and 6 months. If nontreponemal antibody titers have not declined fourfold by 3 months with primary or secondary syphilis, or by 6 months in early latent syphilis, or if signs or symptoms persist and reinfection has been ruled out, patients should have a CSF examination and be retreated appropriately.

HIV-infected patients should have more frequent follow-up, including serologic testing at 1, 2, 3, 6, 9, and 12 months. In addition to the preceding guidelines for 3 and 6 months, any patient with a fourfold increase in titer at any time should have a CSF examination and be treated with the neurosyphilis regimen unless reinfection can be established as the cause of the increased titer.

Lumbar Puncture in Early Syphilis.—CSF abnormalities are common in adults with early syphilis. Despite the frequency of these CSF findings, very few patients develop neurosyphilis when the treatment regimens described above are used. Therefore, unless clinical signs and symptoms of neurologic involvement (such as optic, auditory, cranial nerve, or meningeal symptoms) exist, lumbar puncture is not recommended for routine evaluation of early syphilis. This recommendation also applies to immunocompromised and HIV-infected patients since no clear data currently show that these patients need increased therapy.

All syphilis patients should be counseled concerning the risks of HIV and should be encouraged to be tested for HIV.

Late Latent Syphilis of More Than 1 Year's Duration, Gummas, and Cardiovascular Syphilis. All patients should have a thorough clinical examination. Ideally, all patients with syphilis of more than 1 year's duration should have a cerebrospinal fluid (CSF) examination; however, performance of lumbar puncture can be individualized. In older asymptomatic individuals, the yield of lumbar puncture is likely to be low; however, CSF examination is clearly indicated in the following specific situations:

- Neurologic signs or symptoms
- Treatment failure
- Serum nontreponemal antibody titer ≥1:32
- Other evidence of active syphilis (aortitis, gumma, iritis)
- Nonpenicillin therapy planned
- Positive HIV antibody test results

NOTE: If CSF examination is performed and reveals findings consistent with neurosyphilis, patients should be treated for neurosyphilis (see next section). Some experts also treat cardiovascular syphilis patients with a neurosyphilis regimen.

Recommended Regimen.—***Benzathine penicillin*** *G.* 7.2

million units total, administered as 3 doses of 2.4 million units IM, given 1 week apart for 3 consecutive weeks.

Follow-Up.—Quantitative nontreponemal serologic tests should be repeated at 6 months and 12 months. If titers increase fourfold, if an initially high titer (≥1:32) fails to decrease, or if the patient has signs or symptoms attributable to syphilis, the patient should be evaluated for neurosyphilis and retreated appropriately.

HIV Testing.—All syphilis patients should be counseled concerning the risks of HIV and should be encouraged to be tested for HIV antibody.

Neurosyphilis. Central nervous system disease may occur during any stage of syphilis. Clinical evidence of neurologic involvement (e.g., optic and auditory symptoms, cranial nerve palsies) warrants CSF examination.

Recommended Regimen.—***Aqueous crystalline penicillin*** *G,* 12–24 million units administered 2–4 million units every 4 hours IV, for 10–14 days.

Alternative Regimen (if outpatient compliance can be ensured).—***Procaine penicillin*** 2.4 million units IM daily, **and** ***Probenecid*** 500 mg orally 4 times a day, both for 10–14 days. Many authorities recommend addition of *benzathine penicillin G.* 2.4 million units IM weekly for three doses after completion of these neurosyphilis treatment regimens. No systematically collected data have evaluated therapeutic alternatives to penicillin. Patients who cannot tolerate penicillin should be skin tested and desensitized, if necessary, or managed in consultation with an expert.

Follow-Up.—If an initial CSF pleocytosis was present, CSF examination should be repeated every 6 months until the cell count is normal. If it has not decreased at 6 months, or is not normal by 2 years, retreatment should be strongly considered.

HIV Testing.—All syphilis patients should be counseled concerning the risks of HIV and should be encouraged to be tested for HIV antibody.

Syphilis in Pregnancy

Screening.—Pregnant women should be screened early in pregnancy. Seropositive pregnant women should be considered infected unless treatment history and sequential serologic antibody titers are showing an appropriate response. In populations in which prenatal care utilization is not optimal, patients should be screened, and if necessary, treatment provided at the time pregnancy is detected. In areas of high syphilis prevalence, or in patients at high risk, screening should be repeated in the third trimester and again at delivery.

Treatment.—Patients should be treated with the **penicillin** regimen appropriate for the woman's stage of syphilis. Tetracycline and doxycycline are contraindicated in pregnancy. Erythromycin should not be used because of the high risk of failure to cure infection in the fetus. Pregnant women with histories of penicillin allergy should first be carefully questioned regarding the validity of the history. If necessary, they should then be skin tested and either treated with penicillin or referred for desensitization. Women who are treated in the second half of pregnancy are at risk for **premature labor** or **fetal distress** (or both) if their treatment precipitates a Jarisch-Herxheimer reaction. They should be advised to seek medical attention after treatment if they notice any change in fetal movements or have any contractions. Stillbirth is a rare complication of treatment; however, since therapy is necessary to prevent further fetal damage, this concern should not delay treatment.

Follow-Up.—Monthly follow-up is mandatory so that retreatment can be given if needed. The antibody response should be the same as for nonpregnant patients.

HIV Testing.—All syphilis patients should be counseled concerning the risks of HIV and should be encouraged to be tested for HIV antibody.

Congenital Syphilis

Who Should Be Evaluated.—Infants should be evaluated if they were born to seropositive (nontreponemal test confirmed by treponemal test) women who:

- Have untreated syphilis; ***or***
- Were treated for syphilis less than 1 month **before** delivery; ***or***
- Were treated for syphilis during pregnancy with a nonpenicillin regimen; ***or***
- Did not have the expected decrease in nontreponemal antibody titers after treatment for syphilis; ***or***
- Do not have a well-documented history of treatment for syphilis; ***or***

- Were treated but had insufficient serologic follow-up during pregnancy to assess disease activity.

An infant should not be released from the hospital until the serologic status of the infant's mother is known.

Evaluation of the Infant.—The clinical and laboratory evaluation of infants born to women described should include:

- A thorough physical examination for evidence of congenital syphilis
- Nontreponemal antibody titer
- CSF analysis for cells, protein, and VDRL
- Long bone x-ray examination
- Other tests as clinically indicated (e.g., chest x-ray examination)
- If possible, FTA-ABS on the purified 19S-IgM fraction of serum (e.g., separation by Isolab columns)

Therapy Decisions.—Infants should be treated if they have:

- Any evidence of active disease (physical or x-ray examination); ***or***
- A reactive CSF-VDRL; ***or***
- An abnormal CSF finding (white blood cell count $>5/mm^3$ or protein >50 mg/dl)* regardless of CSF serology; ***or***
- Quantitative nontreponemal serologic titers that are fourfold (or greater) higher than their mother's; ***or***
- Positive FTA-ABS-19S-IgM antibody, if performed.

Even if the evaluation is normal, infants should be treated if their mothers have untreated syphilis or evidence of relapse or reinfection after treatment. Infants, who meet the criteria listed in "Who Should be Evaluated" but are not fully evaluated, should be assumed to be infected and should be treated.

Treatment.—Treatment should consist of: 100,000–150,000 units/kg of **aqueous crystalline penicillin G daily** (administered as 50,000 units/kg IV every 8–12 hours) *or* 50,000 units/kg of **procaine penicillin daily** (administered once IM) for 10–14 days. If more than 1 day of therapy is missed, the entire course **should** be restarted. All symptomatic neonates should also have an ophthalmologic examination.

*In the immediate newborn period, interpretation of these tests may be difficult; normal values vary with gestational age and are higher in preterm infants. Other causes of elevated values should also be considered. However, *when an infant is being evaluated for congenital syphilis*, the infant should be treated if test results cannot exclude infection.

Infants who meet the criteria listed in "Who Should be Evaluated," but who after evaluation do not meet the criteria listed in "Therapy Decisions," **are at low risk for congenital syphilis. If their mothers were treated with erythromycin during pregnancy,** or if close follow-up cannot be **assured,** they should be treated with **benzathine penicillin G,** 50,000 units/kg IM as a one-time dose.

Follow-Up.—Seropositive untreated infants must be closely followed at 1, 2, 3, 6, and 12 months of age. In the absence of infection, nontreponemal antibody titers should be decreasing by 3 months of age and should have disappeared by 6 months of age. If these titers are found to be stable or increasing, the child should be reevaluated and fully treated. Additionally, in the absence of infection, treponemal antibodies may be present up to 1 year. If they are present beyond 1 year, the infant should be treated for congenital syphilis.

Treated infants should also be observed to ensure decreasing nontreponemal antibody titers; these should have disappeared by 6 months of age. Treponemal tests should not be used, since they may remain positive despite effective therapy if the child was infected. Infants with documented CSF pleocytosis should be reexamined every 6 months or until the cell count is normal. If the cell count is still abnormal after 2 years, or if a downward trend is not present at each examination, the infant should be retreated. The CSF-VDRL should also be checked at 6 months; if it is still reactive, the infant should be retreated.

Therapy of Older Infants and Children.—After the newborn period, children discovered to have syphilis should have a CSF examination to rule out congenital syphilis. Any child who is thought to have congenital syphilis or who has neurologic involvement should be treated with 200,000–300,000 units/kg/day of **aqueous crystalline penicillin G** (administered as 50,000 units/kg every 4–6 hours) for 10–14 days. Older children with definite acquired syphilis and a normal neurologic examination may be treated with **benzathine penicillin G,** 50,000 units/kg IM, up to the adult dose of 2.4 million units. Children with a history of penicillin allergy should be skin tested and, if necessary, desensitized. Follow-up should be performed as described previously.

HIV Testing.—In cases of congenital syphilis, the mother should be counseled concerning the risks of HIV and should be encouraged to be tested for HIV; if her test results are positive, the infant should be referred for follow-up.

Syphilis in HIV-Infected Patients

Diagnosis

- All sexually active patients with syphilis should be encouraged to be counseled and tested for HIV because of the frequency of association of the two diseases and the implications for clinical assessment and management.
- Neurosyphilis should be considered in the differential diagnosis of neurologic disease in HIV-infected persons.
- When clinical findings suggest that syphilis is present but serologic tests are negative or confusing, alternative tests, such as biopsy of lesions, dark-field examination, and direct fluorescent antibody staining of lesion material, should be used.
- In cases of congenital syphilis, the mother should be encouraged to be counseled and tested for HIV; if her test results are positive, the infant should be referred for follow-up.

Treatment and Follow-Up

- Penicillin regimens should be used whenever possible for all stages of syphilis in HIV-infected patients. Skin testing to confirm penicillin allergy may be used if minor and major determinants are available. However, data on its use in HIV-infected individuals are inadequate. Patients may be desensitized and treated with penicillin.
- No change in therapy for early syphilis for HIV-coinfected patients is recommended. However, some authorities advise CSF examination or treatment (or both) with a regimen appropriate for neurosyphilis for all patients coinfected with syphilis and HIV, regardless of the clinical stage of syphilis. In all cases, careful follow-up is necessary to ensure adequacy of treatment.
- HIV-infected patients treated for syphilis should be followed up clinically and with quantitative nontreponemal serologic tests (VDRL, RPR) at 1, 2, 3, 6, 9, and 12 months after treatment. Patients with early syphilis whose titers increase or fail to decrease (see section on Follow-Up, Early Syphilis) fourfold within 6 months should undergo CSF examination and be retreated. In such patients CSF abnormalities could be due to HIV-related infection, neurosyphilis, or both. STD clinics and other providers of STD treatment should ensure adequate follow-up.

Management of Patients With Histories of Penicillin Allergy.—Currently, no proved alternative therapies to penicillin are available for treating patients with neurosyphilis, congenital syphilis, or syphilis in pregnancy. Therefore, skin testing—with desensitization, if indicated—is recommended for these patients.

Genital Herpes Simplex Virus Infections

Genital herpes is a viral disease that may be chronic and recurring and for which no known cure exists. Systemic acyclovir treatment provides partial control of the symptoms and signs of herpes episodes; it accelerates healing but does not eradicate the infection nor affect the subsequent risk, frequency, or severity of recurrences after the drug is discontinued. Topical therapy with acyclovir is substantially less effective than therapy with the oral drug.

First Clinical Episode of Genital Herpes

Recommended Regimen.—*Acyclovir,* 200 mg orally 5 times a day for 7–10 days or until clinical resolution occurs.

First Clinical Episode of Herpes Proctitis

Recommended Regimen.—*Acyclovir,* 400 mg orally 5 times a day for 10 days or until clinical resolution occurs.

Inpatient Therapy. For patients with severe disease or complications necessitating hospitalization

Recommended Regimen.—*Acyclovir,* 5 mg/kg body weight IV every 8 hours for 5–7 days or until clinical resolution occurs (encephalitis, pneumonitis, and/or hepatitis), acyclovir administered IV is probably of value. Among pregnant women without life-threatening disease, systemic acyclovir treatment ***should not*** be used for recurrent genital herpes episodes or as suppressive therapy to prevent reactivation near term.

Perinatal Infections. Most mothers of infants who acquire neonatal herpes lack histories of clinically evident genital herpes. The risk of transmission to the neonate from an infected mother is highest among women with primary herpes infection near the time of delivery, and it is low among women with recurrent herpes. The results of viral cultures during pregnancy do not predict viral shedding at the time of delivery; such cultures are not routinely indicated.

At the onset of labor, all women should be examined and carefully questioned about symptoms. Women without symptoms or signs of genital herpes infection or prodrome may have vaginal deliveries. For women who have a history of genital herpes or who have a sex partner with genital herpes, cultures of the birth canal at delivery may be helpful in decisions about neonatal management. Cultures and careful observation are indicated for infants delivered through an infected birth canal (proved by culture or presumed by observation of lesions). Although data are limited concerning the use of acyclovir for asymptomatic infants, some experts presumptively treat infants who were exposed to herpes simplex virus (HSV) at delivery. Herpes cultures should be obtained from infants before therapy; positive cultures obtained 24–48 hours or more after birth indicate active viral infection.

Counseling and Management of Sex Partners.—Patients with genital herpes should be told about the natural history of their disease, with emphasis on the potential for recurrent episodes. Patients should be advised to abstain from sexual activity while lesions are present. Sexual transmission of HSV has been documented during periods without recognized lesions. Suppressive treatment with oral acyclovir reduces the frequency of recurrences but does not totally eliminate viral shedding. Genital herpes and other diseases causing genital ulcers have been associated with an increased risk of acquiring HIV infections; therefore, condoms should be used during all sexual exposures. If sex partners of patients with genital herpes have genital lesions, they may benefit from evaluation; however, evaluation of asymptomatic partners is of little value in preventing transmission of HSV.

The risk of neonatal infection should be explained to all patients—male and female—with genital herpes. Women of childbearing age with genital herpes should be advised to inform their clinicians of their history during any future pregnancy.

Infections of Epithelial Surfaces

Genital Warts

Exophytic genital and anal warts are caused by certain types (most frequently types 6 and 11) of human papillomavirus (HPV). Other types sometimes present in the anogenital region (most commonly types 16, 18, and 31) have been found to be strongly associated with genital dysplasia and carcinoma. For this reason biopsy is needed in all instances of atypical, pigmented, or persistent warts. All women with anogenital warts should have an annual Pap smear.

Some subclinical HPV infections may be detected by Pap

smear and colposcopy. Application of acetic acid may also indicate otherwise subclinical lesions, but false-positive test results occur. Tests for the detection of HPV-DNA are now widely available. The clinical use of these tests in managing individual patients is not known. Therefore therapeutic decisions should not be made on the basis of these HPV-DNA tests.

No therapy has been shown to eradicate HPV. HPV has been demonstrated in adjacent tissue after laser treatment of HPV-associated cervical intraepithelial neoplasia and after attempts to eliminate subclinical HPV by extensive laser vaporization of the anogenital area. The benefit of treating patients with subclinical HPV infection has not been demonstrated, and recurrence is common. The effect of genital wart treatment on HPV transmission and the natural history of HPV are unknown. ***Therefore, the goal of treatment is removal of exophytic warts and the amelioration of signs and symptoms, not the eradication of HPV.***

Expensive therapies, toxic therapies, and procedures that result in scarring should be avoided. Sex partners should be examined for evidence of warts. Patients with anogenital warts should be made aware that they are contagious to uninfected sex partners. The use of condoms is recommended to help reduce transmission.

In most clinical situations, cryotherapy with liquid nitrogen or cryoprobe is the treatment of choice for external genital and perianal warts. Cryotherapy is nontoxic, does not require anesthesia, and—if used properly—does not result in scarring. Podophyllin, trichloroacetic acid, and electrodesiccation/electrocautery are alternative therapies. Treatment with interferon is not recommended because of its relatively low efficacy, high incidence of toxicity, and high cost.

The carbon dioxide laser and conventional surgery are useful in the management of extensive warts, particularly for patients who have not responded to cryotherapy; these alternatives are not appropriate for limited lesions. Like more cost-effective treatments, these therapies do not eliminate HPV and often are associated with the recurrence of clinical cases.

Pregnant Patients and Perinatal Infections. Cesarean delivery for prevention of transmission of HPV infection to the neonate is not indicated. In rare instances, however, cesarean delivery may be indicated for women with genital warts if the pelvic outlet is obstructed or if vaginal delivery would result in excessive bleeding.

Genital papillary lesions have a tendency to proliferate and to become friable during pregnancy. Many experts advocate removal of visible warts during pregnancy, although data on this subject are limited.

HPV can cause laryngeal papillomatosis in infants. The route of transmission (transplacental, birth canal, or postnatal) is unknown; therefore, the preventive value of cesarean delivery is unknown. The perinatal transmission rate is also unknown, although it must be very low, given the relatively high prevalence of genital warts and the rarity of laryngeal papillomas. Neither routine HPV screening tests nor cesarean delivery is indicated to prevent transmission of HPV infection to the neonate.

Treatment Recommendations

External Genital/Perianal Warts

Recommended Regimen.—**Cryotherapy with liquid nitrogen or cryoprobe.**

Alternative Regimen.—*Podophyllin* 10%–25% in compound tincture of benzoin. Limit the total volume of podophyllin solution applied to <0.5 mL per treatment session. Thoroughly wash off in 1–4 hours. Treat <10 cm^2 per session. Repeat applications at weekly intervals. Mucosal warts are more likely to respond than highly keratinized warts on the penile shaft, buttocks, and pubic areas. ***Contraindicated in pregnancy.***

Trichloroacetic acid (80%–90%). Apply only to warts; powder with talc or sodium bicarbonate (baking soda) to remove unreacted acid. Repeat application at weekly intervals.

Electrodesiccation/electrocautery. Electrodesiccation is contraindicated in patients with cardiac pacemakers, or for lesions proximal to the anal verge. Extensive or refractory disease should be referred to an expert.

Cervical Warts

Recommended Regimen.—For women with cervical warts, dysplasia must be excluded before treatment is begun. Management should therefore be carried out in consultation with an expert.

Vaginal Warts

Recommended Regimen.—*Cryotherapy* with liquid nitrogen. (The use of a cryoprobe in the vagina is not recommended because of the risk of vaginal perforation and fistula formation.)

Alternative Regimen.—*Trichloroacetic acid* (80%–90%). Apply only to warts; powder with talc or sodium bicarbonate (baking soda) to remove unreacted acid. Repeat application at weekly intervals.

Podophyllin 10%–25% in compound tincture of benzoin. Treatment area must be dry before speculum is removed. Treat $<2\ cm^2$ per session. Repeat application at weekly intervals. ***Contraindicated in pregnancy.*** Extensive or refractory disease should be referred to an expert.

Urethral Meatus Warts

Recommended Regimen.—**Cryotherapy** with liquid nitrogen.

Alternative Regimen.—*Podophyllin* 10%–25% in compound tincture of benzoin. Treatment area must be dry before contact with normal mucosa, and podophyllin must be washed off in 1–2 hours. ***Contraindicated in pregnancy.*** Extensive or refractory disease should be referred to an expert.

Anal Warts

Recommended Regimen.—**Cryotherapy** with liquid nitrogen. Extensive or refractory disease should be referred to an expert.

Gonococcal Infections

Treatment of gonococcal infections in the United States is influenced by the following trends: (1) the spread of infections due to antibiotic-resistant *Neisseria gonorrhoeae,* including penicillinase-producing *N. gonorrhoeae* (PPNG), tetracycline-resistant *N. gonorrhoeae* (TRNG), and strains with chromosomally mediated resistance to multiple antibiotics; (2) the high frequency of chlamydial infections in persons with gonorrhea; (3) recognition of the serious complications of chlamydial and gonococcal infections; and (4) the absence of a fast, inexpensive, and highly accurate test for chlamydial infection.

All cases of gonorrhea should be diagnosed or confirmed by culture to facilitate antimicrobial susceptibility testing. The susceptibility of *N. gonorrhoeae* to antibiotics is likely to change after a period of time in any locality. Therefore gonorrhea control programs should include a system of regular antibiotic sensitivity testing of a surveillance sample of *N. gonorrhoeae* isolates as well as all isolates associated with treatment failure.

Because of the wide spectrum of antimicrobial therapies effective against *N. gonorrhoeae,* these guidelines are *not* intended to be a comprehensive list of all possible treatment regimens.

Treatment of Gonococcal Infections in Pregnancy.—Cultures of pregnant women should be taken and tested for *N. gonorrhoeae* (and also for *Chlamydia trachomatis* and syphilis) at the first prenatal care visit. For women at high risk of STD, a second culture for gonorrhea (as well as tests for chlamydia and syphilis) should be obtained late in the third trimester.

Recommended Regimen.—*Ceftriaxone,* 250 mg IM once; ***plus*** *Erythromycin* base* 500 mg orally 4 times a day for 7 days.

Pregnant women allergic to β-lactams should be treated with **spectinomycin,** 2 g IM once ***(followed by*** **erythromycin).** Follow-up cervical and rectal cultures for *N. gonorrhoeae* should be obtained 4–7 days after treatment is completed.

Ideally, pregnant women with gonorrhea should be treated for chlamydia on the basis of chlamydial diagnostic studies. If chlamydial diagnostic testing is not available, treatment for chlamydia should be given. Tetracyclines (including doxycycline) and the quinolones are contraindicated in pregnancy because of possible adverse effects on the fetus. Treatments for pregnant patients with chlamydial infection, acute salpingitis, and disseminated gonorrhea in pregnancy are described in respective sections.

Gonococcal Infections of Infants

Treatment of Infants Born to Mothers With Gonococcal Infection.—Infants born to mothers with untreated gonorrhea are at high risk of infection (e.g., ophthalmia and disseminated gonococcal infection) [DGI] and should be treated with a single injection of *ceftriaxone* (50 mg/kg IV or IM, not to exceed 125 mg). Ceftriaxone should be given cautiously to hyperbilirubinemic infants, especially premature infants. Topical prophylaxis for neonatal ophthalmia is not adequate treatment for documented infections of the eye or other sites.

Treatment of Infants With Gonococcal Infection.—Infants with documented gonococcal infections at any site (e.g., eye) should be evaluated for DGI. This evaluation should include a careful physical examination, especially of the joints, as well as blood and CSF cultures. Infants with gonococcal ophthalmia or

***Erythromycin** stearate (500 mg) or **erythromycin ethylsuccinate** (800 mg) or equivalent may be substituted for erythromycin base.

DGI should be treated for 7 days (10 to 14 days if meningitis is present) with one of the following regimens.

Recommended Regimen.—*Ceftriaxone* 25–50 mg/kg/day IV or IM in a single daily dose, ***or,*** *Cefotaxime* 25 mg/kg IV or IM every 12 hours.

Alternative Regimen.—Limited data suggest that uncomplicated gonococcal ophthalmia among infants may be cured with a single injection of *ceftriaxone* (50 mg/kg up to 125 mg). A few experts use this regimen for children who have no clinical or laboratory evidence of disseminated disease.

If the gonococcal isolate is proved to be susceptible to penicillin, **crystalline penicillin G** may be given. The dose is 100,000 units/kg/day given in two equal doses (four equal doses per day for infants more than 1 week old). The dose should be increased to 150,000 units/kg/day for meningitis.

Infants with gonococcal ophthalmia should receive eye irrigations with buffered saline solutions until discharge has cleared. Topical antibiotic therapy alone is inadequate. Simultaneous infection with *C. trachomatis* has been reported and should be considered for patients who do not respond satisfactorily. Therefore the mother and the infant should be tested for chlamydial infection.

Prevention of Ophthalmia Neonatorum

Instillation of a prophylactic agent into the eyes of all newborn infants is recommended to prevent gonococcal ophthalmia neonatorum and is required by law in most states. Although all regimens listed below effectively prevent gonococcal eye disease, their efficacy in preventing chlamydial eye disease is not clear. Furthermore, they do not eliminate nasopharyngeal colonization with *C. trachomatis*. Treatment of gonococcal and chlamydial infections in pregnant women is the best method for preventing neonatal gonococcal and chlamydial disease.

Recommended Regimen.—*Erythromycin* (0.5%) ophthalmic ointment, once, ***or,*** *Tetracycline* (1%) ophthalmic ointment, once, ***or,*** *Silver nitrate* (1%) aqueous solution, once.

One of these should be instilled into the eyes of every neonate as soon as possible after delivery, and definitely within 1 hour after birth. Single-use tubes or ampules are preferable to multiple-use tubes.

The efficacy of tetracycline and erythromycin in the prevention of tetracycline-resistant *N. gonorrhoeae* and penicillinase-producing *N. gonorrhoeae* ophthalmia is unknown, although both are probably effective because of the high concentrations of drug in these preparations. Bacitracin is ***not*** recommended.

Chlamydial Infections

Culture and nonculture methods for diagnosis of *C. trachomatis* infection are now available. Appropriate use of these diagnostic tests is strongly encouraged, especially for screening asymptomatic high-risk women in whom infection would otherwise be undetected. However, in clinical settings where testing for chlamydia is not routine or available, treatment often is prescribed on the basis of clinical diagnosis or as cotreatment for gonorrhea (see Gonococcal Infections). In clinical settings periodic surveys should be performed to determine local chlamydial prevalence in patients with gonorrhea. Priority groups for chlamydia testing, if resources are limited, are high-risk pregnant women, adolescents, and women with multiple sexual partners.

Results of chlamydial tests should be interpreted with care. The sensitivity of all currently available laboratory tests for *C. trachomatis* is substantially less than 100%; thus false-negative tests are possible. Although the specificity of nonculture tests has improved substantially, false-positive test results may still occur with nonculture tests. Persons with chlamydial infections may remain asymptomatic for extended periods of time.

Treatment of C. trachomatis *in Pregnancy*

Pregnant women should undergo diagnostic testing for *C. trachomatis, N. gonorrhoeae,* and syphilis, if possible, at their first prenatal visit and, for women at high risk, during the third trimester. Risk factors for chlamydial disease during pregnancy include young age (<25 years), past history or presence of other STD, a new sex partner within the preceding 3 months, and multiple sex partners. Ideally, pregnant women with gonorrhea should be treated for chlamydia on the basis of diagnostic studies, but if chlamydial testing is not available, treatment should be given because of the high likelihood of coinfection.

Recommended Regimen.—*Erythromycin* base, 500 mg orally 4 times a day for 7 days. If this regimen is not tolerated, the following regimens are recommended.

Alternative Regimen.—*Erythromycin* base, 250 mg orally 4 times a day for 14 days, ***or,*** *Erythromycin ethylsuccinate,* 800 mg orally 4 times a day for 7 days, ***or,*** **Erythromycin ethylsuccinate,** 400 mg orally 4 times a day for 14 days.

Alternative if Erythromycin Cannot Be Tolerated.—*Amoxicillin,* 500 mg orally three times a day for 7 days (limited data exist concerning this regimen). *Erythromycin estolate* is contraindicated during pregnancy, since drug-related hepatoxicity can result.

Sex Partners of Patients With C. trachomatis *Infections*

Sex partners of patients who have *C. trachomatis* infection should be tested and treated for *C. trachomatis* if their contact was within 30 days of onset of symptoms. If testing is not available, they should be treated with the appropriate antimicrobial regimen.

Bacterial Vaginosis

Bacterial vaginosis (BV) (formerly called nonspecific vaginitis, *Haemophilus*-associated vaginitis, or *Gardnerella*-associated vaginitis) is the clinical result of alterations in the vaginal microflora. Clinical diagnosis is made when three or four criteria (homogeneous discharge, pH >4.5, positive amine odor test, or presence of clue cells) are present. Diagnosis can also be made from Gram's stain. Asymptomatic infections are common. Many authorities do not recommend treatment for asymptomatic infection.

Treatment of Male Partners.—No clinical counterpart of BV is recognized in the male, and treatment of the male sex partner has not been shown to be beneficial for the patient or the male partner.

BV in Pregnant Patients.—In pregnancy, recent studies suggest that BV may be a factor in premature rupture of membranes and premature delivery; thus close clinical follow-up of pregnant women with BV is essential. These studies require confirmation, however, and intervention studies have not been conducted. Until such studies have been conducted, routine treatment appears to be unnecessary, and treatment of pregnant women with BV should be at the option of the physician.

Metronidazole is contraindicated in the first trimester of pregnancy, and its safety in the rest of pregnancy is not established. Thus treatment with **clindamycin,** 300 mg orally twice daily for 7 days, is recommended.

Ectoparasitic Infections

Pediculosis Pubis

Recommended Regimen.—Permethrin (1%) creme rinse applied to affected area and washed off after 10 minutes, ***or,*** *Pyrethrins* and *piperonyl butoxide* applied to the affected area and washed off after 10 minutes, ***or,*** *Lindane* 1% shampoo applied for 4 minutes and then thoroughly washed off. (Not recommended for pregnant or lactating women.)

Patients should be reevaluated after 1 week if symptoms persist. Retreatment may be necessary if lice are found or eggs are observed at the hair-skin junction.

Sex partners should be treated as above.

Special Considerations. Pediculosis of the eyelashes should be treated by the application of occlusive ophthalmic ointment to the eyelid margins, two times a day for 10 days, to smother lice and nits. Lindane or other drugs should not be applied to the eyes. Clothing or bed linen that may have been contaminated by the patient within the preceding 2 days should be washed and dried by machine (hot cycle in each) or dry cleaned.

Scabies

Recommended Regimen (Adults and Older Children).— Lindane (1%) 1 oz. of lotion or 30 g of cream applied thinly to all areas of the body from the neck down and washed off thoroughly after 8 hours. (Not recommended for pregnant or lactating women.)

Alternative Regimen.—Crotamiton (10%) applied to the entire body from the neck down for two nights and washed off thoroughly 24 hours after the second application. *Infants, Children 2 Years of Age or Less, Pregnant and Lactating Women:* For these groups, lindane is contraindicated. The crotamiton regimen should be used. *Contacts:* Sex partners and close household contacts should be treated as above.

Special Considerations. Pruritus may persist for several weeks after adequate therapy. A single retreatment after 1 week may be appropriate if no clinical improvement occurs. Additional weekly treatments are warranted only if live mites can be demonstrated. Clothing or bed linen that may have been contaminated by the patient within the preceding 2 days should be washed and dried by machine (hot cycle in each) or dry cleaned.

APPENDIX R: DRUGS OF ABUSE: URINE DRUG SCREENS

Various screening techniques are available to detect the presence of medications in a patient. The qualitative thin-layer chromatography with enzyme-multiplied immunoassay (EMIT) confirmation of opiates, cocaine, and benzodiazepines (three areas of TLC weakness) is the most commonly ordered initial urine drug test in university and large private hospitals. The comprehensive quantitative drug test is useful once the qualitative test identifies a particular substance in the patient's urine sample. Alcohol and marijuana are not routinely analyzed on these tests. Alcohol is detected best in the blood. Both of these chemicals may be requested and added onto the standard TLC-EMIT panel used at your hospital.

TABLE R–1.
Screening Criteria for Drugs of Abuse

Antepartum hemorrhage
History of IV drug use
Preterm labor
Preterm premature rupture of membranes
Pregnancy-induced hypertension
Bizarre behavior
No prenatal care
Tattoos
History of hepatitis
Unexplained seizure
Obtundation

TABLE R–2.

Drug of Abuse Screen, Qualitative

Technique:	Screen: Thin-layer chromatography, enzyme-multiplied immunoassay Confirm: TLC, EMIT, HPLC, GLC, GCMS
Specimen required:	50 mL urine
Analytic time:	2–4 hr
Day(s) test set up:	Daily Available stat
Normal test values:	None detected

This rapid qualitative analysis is performed on urine and is designed for the detection of drugs in the overdose situation. The drugs listed below are detected as either their parent compound or their urinary metabolite.

Analyses Performed

- Amphetamines
  - Amphetamine
  - Methamphetamine
- Antidepressants
  - Amitriptyline (Elavil)
  - Amoxepin
  - Desipramine (Norpramin)
  - Doxepin (Sinequan)
  - Imipramine (Tofranil)
  - Nortriptyline (Aventyl)
- Antihistamines
  - Diphenhydramine (Benadryl)
  - Dimenhydrinate (Dramamine)
- Narcotics
  - Codeine
  - Hydrocodone
  - Hydromorphone
  - Meperidine (Demerol)
  - Methadone (Dolophine)
  - Morphine (Heroin)
  - Norpropoxyphene
  - Pentazocine (Talwin)
  - Propoxyphene (Darvon)
- Phenothiazines (undifferentiated)
- Sedatives and hypnotics
  - Ethchlorvynol (Placidyl)

- Ephedrine (Isupres)
- Pseudoephedrine
- Phenylpropanolamine (Dietac)

Barbiturates

- Amobarbital (Amytal)
- Butabarbital (Butabarb)
- Butalbital
- Pentobarbital (Nembutal)
- Phenobarbital (Luminal)
- Secobarbital (Seconal)

Benzodiazepines (undifferentiated)

Cardiacs

Lidocaine (Xylocaine)

Quinidine/quinine

- Glutethimide (Doriden)
- Meprobamate (Equanil)
- Methaqualone (Quaalude)

Miscellaneous Agents

- Cocaine (as benzoylecgonine)
- Dextromethorphan
- Phencyclidine (PCP)
- Phentermine
- Phenytoin (Dilantin)
- Strychnine

Test code: DAUSC

EMIT = enzyme-multiplied immunoassay; GCMS = gas chromatography–mass spectrometry; GLC = gas-liquid chromatography; HPLC = high-pressure liquid chromatography; TLC = thin-layer chromatography;

TABLE R–3.

Drug Comprehensive Panel, Quantitative* †

Technique:	Screen: Thin-layer chromatography, spectrophotometric, EMIT Confirm: TLC, EMIT, HPLC, GLC, GCMS
Specimen required:	75 mL random urine; 15 mL serum and gastric contents (if available). *Do not use serum separator tubes.* Consultation with the attending physician is desirable. Blood and urine are required for complete analysis. If only blood is submitted, only the drugs marked by an asterisk can be detected. If only urine is submitted, all classes of drugs will be detected as either the parent compound or its urinary metabolite.
Analytic time:	Positive result: dependent on the number of drugs detected None detected: Results within 3 hours
Day(s) test set up:	Daily Available stat
Normal test values:	None detected This analysis is particularly valuable when drug overdose is possible or suspected, but the causative agent is unknown and other data available to the physician are insufficient to permit definite treatment. The study includes qualitative analysis for the types of drugs listed below and blood quantitations of the drugs marked with an asterisk (*).

ANALYSES PERFORMED

Amphetamines	Narcotics
Amphetamine	Codeine
Methamphetamine	Hydrocodone
Analgesics	Hydromorphone
*Acetaminophen (Tylenol)	Meperidine (Demerol)
*Salicylate (Aspirin)	Methadone (Dolophine)
Antidepressants	Morphine (heroin)
Amitriptyline (Elavil)	Norpropoxyphene
Amoxepin	Pentazocine (Talwin)
Desipramine (Norpramin)	Propoxyphene (Darvon) and metabolite

Doxepin (Sinequan)
Imipramine (Tofranil)
Maprotiline (Ludiomil)
Nortriptyline (Aventyl)

Antihistamines
- Diphenhydramine (Benadryl)
- Dimenhydrinate (Dramamine)
- Ephedrine (Isupres)/pseudoephedrine
- Methapyrilene
- Phenylpropanolamine (Dietac)
- Pyrilamine

Barbiturates
- *Amobarbital (Amytal)
- *Butabarbital (Butabarb)/Butalbital
- *Pentobarbital (Nembutal)
- *Phenobarbital (Luminal)
- *Secobarbital (Seconal)
- Benzodiazepines
- *Chlordiazepoxide (Librium)
- *Diazepam (Valium)/and metabolite
- Oxazepam

Cardiacs
- Lidocaine (Xylocaine)
- Quinidine/quinine

Phenothiazines (undifferentiated unless parent present)
- Chlorpromazine (Thorazine)
- Thioridazine (Mellaril)
- Trifluoperazine (Stelazine)
- Trifluorpromazine
- Trimeprazine
- Sedatives and hypnotics
- *Carisoprodol (Soma)
- *Ethchlorvynol (Placidyl)
- Ethinamate (Valmid)
- *Glutethimide (Doriden)
- Mebutamate
- *Meprobamate (Equanil)
- *Methaqualone (Quaalude)
- *Methocarbamol (Robaxin)
- *Methyprylon (Noludar)

Miscellaneous Agents
- Cocaine (as benzoylecgonine)
- Dextromethorphan (Nyquil)
- *Ethanol
- Phencyclidine (PCP)
- Phentermine
- Strychnine

Test code: COMADS

*Modified from *Toxicology Laboratory* Handbook. Irvine, California, University of California at Irvine Medical Center.

†EMIT = enzyme-multiplied immunoassay; GCMS = gas chromatography–mass spectrometry; GLC = gas-liquid chromatography; HPLC = high-pressure liquid chromatography; TLC = thin-layer chromatography.

TABLE R–4.

Detection Time Guide for Drugs in Urine*

Interpretation of detection time must take into account variability of urine specimens, drug metabolism and half-life, the patient's physical condition, fluid intake, and method and frequency of ingestion. The following are general guidelines only and apply to the commonly used TLC and EMIT confirmation screens for drugs of abuse.

Drug	Sensitivities Cutoff Values	Approximate Detection Time
Alcohol	20 mg/dL	
Amphetamines	300 ng/dL	2 days
Barbiturates	300 ng/mL	Short-acting (i.e., secobarbital), 1 day Long-acting (i.e., phenobarbital), 2–3 weeks
Benzodiazepines	300 ng/mL	3 days if therapeutic dose ingested
Cocaine	300 ng/mL	Metabolite detectable for 2 to 4 days
Methadone	300 ng/mL	Approximately 3 days
Methaqualone	300 ng/mL	14 days
Opiates	300 ng/mL	2 days
Phencyclidine	75 ng/mL	Approximately 8 days
Propoxyphene	300 ng/mL	6 hr to 2 days
THC (marijuana)	100 ng/mL	

*Modified from *Toxicology Laboratory Handbook.* Irvine, California, University of California at Irvine Medical Center.

APPENDIX S: DRUG USE DURING PREGNANCY: MATERNAL AND EMBRYONIC EFFECTS

TABLE S–1.
Frequency of Cocaine and Alcohol Use With Other Substances (in Percent)*†

Alcohol	
T's and blues	53
Heroin	29
Cocaine	19
Methamphetamine	7
Total	19
Cocaine	
Heroin	54
Methamphetamine	12
T's and blues	12
Total	21

*From Cunningham FG, MacDonald PC, Gant NF (eds): *Williams' Obstetrics,* ed 17. Norwalk, Conn, Appleton & Lange, 1989. Used by permission.
†T's and blues = pentazocine (Talwin) and tripelennamine citrate (pyribenzamine citrate).

TABLE S–2.

Summary of Some Maternal Effects of Social and Illicit Substance Use During Pregnancy*

Substance	Placental Abruption	CNS Damage	Intracranial Hemorrhage	Hepatic or Renal Damage
Alcohol	+	+	—	+
Amphetamines	(+)	+	+	?
Barbiturates	–	+	+	?
Benzodiazepines	–	+	–	?
Cocaine†	+	+	+	+
Codeine	–	+	–	?
Heroin	+	+	+	+
Inhalants	?	+	–	+
LSD	?	+	—	?
Marijuana	–	(–)	—	–
Methadone	+	+	–	+
Methamphetamine	(+)	+	?	?
Morphine	(+)	+	–	+
PCP	?	(+)	(+)	+
Tobacco	+	(–)	–	+
T's and blues†	(+)	(+)	(+)	+

*From Cunningham FG, MacDonald PC, Gant NF (eds): *Williams' Obstetrics*, ed 17. Norwalk, Conn, Appleton & Lange, 1989. Used by permission.

†May cause infarction/embolism; T's and blues = pentazocine (Talwin) and tripelennamine citrate (pyribenzamine citrate).

+, Data conclusive of positive findings.

–, Data conclusive of negative findings.

(+), Data inconclusive but suggestive of positive findings.

(–), Data inconclusive but suggestive of negative findings.

?, Risks are unknown.

TABLE S–3.
Summary of Some Embryofetal Effects of Social and Illicit Substance Use During Pregnancy*

Substance	Growth Retardation	Congenital Anomalies	Withdrawal Syndrome
Alcohol	+	+	+
Amphetamines	+	?(−)	+
Barbiturates	+	?(−)	+
Benzodiazepines	?(+)	?(−)	?(+)
Cocaine	+	+	+
Codeine	?(+)	(−)	+
Heroin	+	−	+
Inhalants	+	+	?(−)
LSD	?	(−)	?(−)
Marijuana	+	−	−
Methadone	+	−	+
Methamphetamine	+	−	+
Morphine	+	(−)	+
PCP	+	?	+
Tobacco	+	−	−
T's and blues†	+	(−)	+

*From Cunningham FG, MacDonald PC, Gant NF (eds): *Williams' Obstetrics,* ed 17. Norwalk, Conn, Appleton & Lange, 1989. Used by permission.
†T's and blues = pentazocine (Talwin) and tripelennamine citrate (pyribenzamine citrate).
+, Data conclusive of positive findings.
−, Data conclusive of negative findings.
(+), Data inconclusive but suggestive of positive findings.
(−), Data inconclusive but suggestive of negative findings.
?, Risks are unknown.

APPENDIX T: DRUG USE DURING PREGNANCY: PERINATAL CHARACTERISTICS

TABLE T–1.

Perinatal Characteristics of Offspring of Women Who Abused Methamphetamines Compared With Control Group*

Characteristics	Methamphetamine (*n* = 52)	Controls (*n* = 52)
Birthweight (g)	2,957	3,295†
Head circumference (cm)	48.1	49.8†
Gestational age (wk)	39.1	39.3†
Any congenital abnormality (%)‡	12	14§

*From Cunningham FG, MacDonald PC, Gant NF (eds): *Williams' Obstetrics*, ed 17. Norwalk, Conn, Appleton & Lange, 1989. Used by permission.
†$P < .05$.
‡Major and minor.
§P = NS.

TABLE T–2.

Perinatal Characteristics of Offspring of Women Who Abused T's and Blues ‖ Compared with Control Group*†

Characteristics	T's and Blues‖ (*n* = 23)	Controls (*n* = 100)
Birthweight (g)	2,752	3,295‡
Head circumference (cm)	32	33.9‡
Gestational age (wk)	38.9	39.3§
Congenital abnormalities (%)	13	6†

*From Cunningham FG, MacDonald PC, Gant NF (eds): *Williams' Obstetrics*, ed 17. Norwalk, Conn, Appleton & Lange, 1989. Used by permission.
†This combination of drugs is a less expensive substitute for heroin
‡$P < .05$.
§P = NS.
‖T's and blues = pentazocine (Talwin) and tripelennamine citrate (pyribenzamine citrate).

APPENDIX U: DEFINITION OF TERMS: STREET NAMES OF DRUGS OF ABUSE*†

Substance	Street Names	
Amphetamine (dextroamphetamine)	AMT	Hearts
	Bam	Lid poppers
	B-bombs	Peaches
	Bennies	Pep pills
	Benz	Purple hearts
	Bombita	Roses
	Brain ticklers*	Sparkle plenties
	Brownies	Splash
	Cartwheels	Speed
	Chalk	Tens
	Copilots	Thrusters
	Crossroads	Uppers, uppies, or ups
	Crystal	West coast turn arounds
	Dexies	Whites
	Fives	
Barbiturates	Blockbusters	Nemmies
	Blues*	Nimby
	Brain ticklers*	Pinks
	Courage pills	Rainbows
	Downers*	Red birds
	Downie	Red devils
	Gangster pills	Reds
	G.B.	Reds and blues
	Goofball	Seggy
	Gorilla pills	Tooies
	Idiot pills	Yellow jackets
	King Kong pills	
Benzodiazepines	Downers*	Vals
	Blues*	
Cocaine	Bernies	Dust
	Burese	Flake
	Candyman*	Heaven dust
	Coke	Lady snow
	Cola	Snow
	Corrine	Star dust
	Crack	
Codeine	Blue velvet	

(Continued.)

Substance	Street Names	
Heroin	Bolsa	H-caps
	Boy	Henry
	Brown stuff	Him
	Caballo	Horse
	Candyman*	Junk
	Cura	Poison
	Duji	Scag
	Dogie	Smack
	Doojie	Tapita
	Dope	Tecata
	Harry	White lady
Lysergic acid diethylamide (LSD)	Acid	LSM
	Beast	Microdot (yellow, blue, white, etc.)
	Big D	Mind detergent
	Blue acid	Orange sunshine
	Chief	Pellets
	Deeda	Purple haze
	Electric Kool-Ade	Tabs
	Ghost	Trips
	Hawk	Window pane
	"L"	
Marijuana	Acapulco gold	Joints
	Baby	Juana
	Bhang	Kif
	Black gunion	Loco weed
	Duby or dooby	Maruamba
	Giggle weed	Mary Jane
	Grass	Pot
	Grefa, greta, grifa, or griffo	Rafe
		Reefer
	Gunjah	Rosa Maria
	Hamp	Skunk
	Hash, hashish, hash oil (extracted from marijuana)	Smoke
		Texas tea
		Yamba
	Herb	
	Hootch	
Methamphetamines	Adam	MDA
	Black beauties	MDMA
	Crank	MDEA
	Ecstasy	Meth
	Eve	Methedrine
	Ice	Crystal
PCP	Angel dust	

*From Cunningham FG, MacDonald PC, Gant NF (eds): *Williams' Obstetrics*, ed 17. Norwalk, Conn, Appleton & Lange, 1989. Used by permission.
†Duplicate street terms are marked with an asterisk.

APPENDIX V: DEFINITION OF TERMS: VITAL STATISTICS*

To aid in the reduction of the number of mothers and infants who die as the result of pregnancy and labor, it is important to know how many such deaths there are in this country each year and in what circumstances. To evaluate these data correctly, a variety of events concerned with pregnancy outcomes have been defined by various agencies:

Birth. This is the complete expulsion or extraction from the mother of a fetus irrespective of whether the umbilical cord has been cut or the placenta is attached. Fetuses weighing less than 500 g usually are not considered as births, but rather as *abortuses,* for purposes of perinatal statistics. In the absence of a birthweight, a body length of 25 cm, crown to heel, is usually equated with 500 g.

Approximately 20 weeks gestational age is commonly considered to be equivalent to 500 g fetal weight; however, a 500 g fetus is more likely to be 22 (menstrual) weeks gestational age.

Birth Rate. The number of births per 1,000 population is the birth rate, or crude birth rate. The birth rate in the United States for the year ending February 1988 was 15.7 (National Center for Health Statistics, 1988).

Fertility Rate. This term refers to the number of live births per 1,000 female population aged 15 through 44 years. In 1987 this was 65.9.

Live Birth. Whenever the infant at or sometime after birth breathes spontaneously or shows any other sign of life such as heartbeat or definite spontaneous movement of voluntary muscles, a live birth is recorded.

Stillbirth. None of the signs of life are present at or after birth.

Neonatal Death. Early neonatal death refers to death of a liveborn infant during the first 7 days after birth. Late neonatal death refers to death after 7 but before 29 days.

Stillbirth Rate. The number of stillborn infants per 1,000 infants born.

Fetal Death Rate. This term is synonymous with stillbirth rate.

Neonatal Mortality Rate. The number of neonatal deaths per 1,000 live births.

Perinatal Mortality Rate. This rate is defined as the number of stillbirths plus neonatal deaths per 1,000 total births.

Low Birthweight. If the first newborn weight obtained after birth is less than 2,500 g, the infant is termed low birthweight.

Term Infant. An infant born anytime after 37 completed (menstrual) weeks of gestation through 42 completed weeks of gestation (260 to 294 days) is considered by most to be a term infant. Such a definition implies that birth at any time within this period is optimal whereas birth before or afterward is not. Such an implication is not warranted. Some infants born between 37 and 38 weeks are at risk of functional prematurity, for example, the development of respiratory distress in the newborn infant of a diabetic mother. In the past, some considered gestation extending past 41 weeks to be postterm; however, any risk to the fetus that might be imposed by remaining in utero until 42 weeks rather than 41 weeks does not appear to be appreciable. Consequently, there is no good reason for distorting the range for term birth to 3 weeks below the mean of 40 weeks but only 1 week beyond the mean.

Preterm or Premature Infant. An infant born before 37 completed weeks has been so classified, although born before 38 completed weeks would seem more appropriate for reasons stated above.

Postterm Infant. An infant born anytime after completion of the 42nd week has been classified by some as being postterm.

Abortus. A fetus or embryo removed or expelled from the uterus during the first half of gestation (20 weeks or less), or weighing less than 500 g, or measuring less than 25 cm is also referred to as an abortus.

Direct Maternal Death. Death of the mother resulting from obstetrical complications of the pregnancy state, labor, or puerperium, and from interventions, omissions, incorrect treatment, or a chain of events resulting from any of the above is considered a direct maternal death. An example is maternal death from exsanguination resulting from rupture of the uterus.

Indirect Maternal Death. An obstetrical death not directly due to obstetrical causes but resulting from previously existing disease, or a disease that developed during pregnancy, labor, or the puerperium, but which was aggravated by the maternal physiological adaptation to pregnancy, is classified as an indirect maternal death. An example is maternal death from complications of mitral stenosis.

Nonmaternal Death. Death of the mother resulting from accidental or incidental causes in no way related to the pregnancy may be classified as a nonmaternal death. An example is death from an automobile accident.

Maternal Death Rate or Maternal Mortality. The number of maternal deaths that result from the reproductive process per 100,000 live births.

*From Cunningham FG, MacDonald PC, Gant NF (eds): *Williams' Obstetrics*, ed 17. Norwalk, Conn, Appleton & Lange, 1989. Used by permission.

APPENDIX W: DEFINITION OF TERMS: SYMBOLS

Symbol	Meaning
$\dot{\bar{\text{I}}}$	one
$\ddot{\bar{\text{II}}}$	two, etc.
$\mu\ell$	microliter
$\pm$	plus or minus
$>$	greater than
$<$	less than
1°	primary
Ψ	psychiatry
$\rightarrow$	to, towards
$\neq$	against, opposite
$\cong$	approximately equal to

Δ	change
[abdominal diagram with x]	location of abdominal findings
+	positive
β	beta
@	at
↑	increased
↓	decreased
♀	female
♂	male
Ⓡ	right
Ⓛ	left
Ⓜ	murmur

Symbol	Meaning
2°	**secondary**
(hand-drawn cross with x)	**location of fetal heart tones**
~	**proportional to**
(hand-drawn stick figure with x)	**location of pulses or reflexes**
( )	**degree**
1:1	**one to one**
—	**negative**

APPENDIX X: DEFINITION OF TERMS: ABBREVIATIONS

A

ā	before
a	arterial
aa	of each; arteries
Ab	abortion
abd	abdomen
ABE	acute bacterial endocarditis
ABG	arterial blood gas
ac	before meals
A/C	assist control
AC	acromioclavicular
ACT	activated clotting time
ACTH	adrenocorticotropic hormone
a.d.	right ear
ADA	American Diabetic Association
ADH	antidiuretic hormone
ad lib	freely, as desired
ADL	activities of daily living
adm	admission
ADP	adenosine diphosphate
adx	adnexa
AF	atrial fibrillation
AFB	acid-fast bacillus
afeb	afebrile
AGE	acute gastroenteritis
+A/G	albumin to globulin ratio
$AgNO_3$	silver nitrate
A/H	auditory hallucinations
AHF	antihemolytic factor
AHFS	American Hospital Formulary Service
AI	aortic insufficiency
AIDS	acquired immunodeficiency syndrome
AK	above the knee
aka	also known as
AKA	above the knee amputation
$AL(OH)_3$	aluminum hydroxide
alk phos	alkaline phosphatase

ALD	alcoholic liver disease
ALL	acute lymphocytic leukemia
ALT	alanine aminotransferase (SGPT)
AMA	against medical advice
amb	ambulate
AML	acute myeloblastic leukemia
amnio	amniocentesis
amp	amputation
amt	amount
ANA	antinuclear antibodies
angio	angiography
anx. neur.	anxiety neurosis
anx. reac.	anxiety reaction
AODM	adult-onset diabetes mellitus
AOM	acute otitis media
A&P	anterior and posterior
AP	anteroposterior
APAP	acetaminophen
Appy	appendectomy
aq	water
AR	aortic regurgitation
ARDS	acute respiratory distress syndrome
ARF	acute renal failure
AROM	artificial rupture of membranes
ARV	alleged rape victim
a.s.	left ear
AS	aortic stenosis
ASA	aspirin
ASAP	as soon as possible
ASAV	alleged sexual assault victim
ASB	asymptomatic bacteriuria
ASCVD	arteriosclerotic cardiovascular disease
ASD	atrial septal defect
ASHD	arteriosclerotic heart disease
ASO	antistreptolysis O
AST	aspartate aminotransferase (SGOT)
at	atrial
ATN	acute tubular necrosis
ATP	adenosine triphosphate
a.u.	aures uterque (each ear)
AV	atrioventricular

A/V	auditory/visual
A/W	alive and well
ax	axillary

B

BBB	bundle branch block
BBBB	bilateral bundle branch block
B&C	board and care
BCC	basal cell carcinoma
BCG	bacillus Calmette-Guérin
BCP	birth control pills
BCS	battered child syndrome
BE	barium enema
be	base excess
BIB	brought in by
BIBPD	brought in by Police Department
BICU	Burn Intensive Care Unit
bid	*bis in die* (twice daily)
BK	below knee
BKA	below the knee amputation
blbs	bilateral breath sounds
blk	block
BM	bowel movement
BMR	basal metabolic rate
BOA	born out of asepsis
BOE	bilateral otitis externa
BOM	bilateral otitis media
BOW	bag of water
BP	blood pressure
BPH	benign prostatic hypertrophy
BPM	beats per minute
BPP	biophysical profile
BR	bed rest
BRBPR	bright red blood per rectum
BRP	bathroom privileges
bs	blood sugar
BS	bowel sounds
B/S	breath sounds
BSA	body surface area
BSO	bilateral salpingo-oophorectomy
BSP	Bromsulphalein

BTL	bilateral tubal ligation
btw	between
BU	Burn Unit
BUN	blood urea nitrogen
BW	birth weight
BWS	battered wife syndrome
Bx	biopsy

C

$\bar{c}$	with
C	centrigrade or Celsius, degree of
C1–C2	first and second cervical
Ca^{++}	calcium
CA	cancer, carcinoma
CABG	coronary artery bypass graft
$CaCl_2$	calcium chloride
$CaCO_3$	calcium carbonate
CAD	coronary artery disease
CAH	congenital adrenal hyperplasia
cap	capsule
cath	catheterization
CBC	complete blood count
CBD	common bile duct
CBDE	common bile duct exploration
CBS	chronic brain syndrome
CC	chief complaint
cc	cubic centimeter
c/c/e	cyanosis, clubbing, edema
CCU	Coronary Care Unit
CDC	Centers for Disease Control
CF	cystic fibrosis
cf	count fingers
CHB	complete heart block
CHD	congenital heart disease
CHF	congestive heart failure
chr	chronic
chr ETOH	chronic alcoholism
circ	circumcision
cis Pt	*cis*-platinum
CK	creatine kinase
CLL	chronic lymphocytic leukemia

cm	centimeter
CML	chronic myelocytic leukemia
CMS	circulation, motion, and sensation
CMV	cytomegalovirus
CNS	central nervous system
C/O	complaints of
CO	cardiac output
CO_2	carbon dioxide
cocci	coccidioidomycosis
COM	chronic otitis media
comp	compound
COPD	chronic obstructive pulmonary disease
CP	cerebral palsy
CPAP	continuous positive airway pressure
CPD	cephalopelvic disproportion
Cpeak	peak compliance
CPK	creatinine phosphokinase; *see* CK
CPR	cardiopulmonary resuscitation
CRF	chronic renal failure
CRIT	hematocrit (hct)
C&S	culture and sensitivity
CS	cesarean section
CSF	cerebrospinal fluid
CST	contraction stress test
Cstat	static compliance
CT	computed tomography
CUS	chronic undifferentiated schizophrenia
CV	cardiovascular
CVA	cerebrovascular accident
CVAT	costovertebral angle tenderness
CVD	cardiovascular disease
CVP	central venous pressure
cx	cervix
CXR	chest x-ray

D

D/C	discontinue
D&C	dilatation and curettage
DCR	dacryocystorhinotomy
DD	differential diagnosis
decel	deceleration

depr neur	depressive neurosis
DFA	diet for age
DI	diabetes insipidus
DIC	disseminated intravascular coagulation
diff	differential count
DIP	distal interphalangeal joint
DJD	degenerative joint disease
DKA	diabetic ketoacidosis
DL&B	direct laryngoscopy and bronchoscopy
D5LR	dextrose 5% Ringer's lactate
DM	diabetes mellitus
DMD	Doctor of Dental Medicine
DNA	deoxyribonucleic acid
DNR	do not resuscitate
D5½NS	5% dextrose and 0.45% N/S
DOA	dead on arrival
DOE	dyspnea on exertion
DPT	diphtheria-pertussis-tetanus immunization
DR	diabetic retinopathy
drsg	dressing
D/S	dextrose in saline
DSD	discharge summary dictated
DSS	dioctyl sodium sulfosuccinate
DT	delerium tremens
DTR	deep tendon reflexes
DU	duodenal ulcer
DUB	dysfunctional uterine bleeding
D5W	5% dextrose in water
D/W	dextrose in water
Dx	diagnosis
DZ	dizygotic (twins)

E

E	esophoria (distance, i.e., 20 ft; 6 m)
E′	esophoria (near, i.e., 14 in.; 33 cm)
EBL	estimated blood loss
ECCE	extracapsular cataract extraction
ECF	extended care facility
ecf	extracellular fluid
ECG	electrocardiogram

ECT	electroconvulsive therapy
EDC	estimated date of confinement (due date)
EEG	electroencephalogram
EENT	eyes, ears, nose, and throat
EFW	estimated fetal weight
e.g.	for example
EGA	estimated gestational age
EICT	external isometric contraction
EKG	electrocardiogram
elix	elixir
EMG	electromyogram
EMI	computed tomography
ENG	electronystagmogram
ENT	ear, nose, and throat
EOMI	extraocular movements intact
EOMs	extraocular movements
eos	eosinophils
EPS	extrapyramidal symptoms
E&R	equal and reactives
ER	Emergency Room
ERE	Emergency Room Emergent
ERN	Emergency Room Nonemergent
ERU	Emergency Room Urgent
ERV	expiratory reserve volume
ESR	erythrocyte sedimentation rate
et	and
(ET)	intermittent esotropia
ET	esotropia (distance)
ET	endotracheal
eth	ethyl alcohol
ETI	endotracheal intubation
ETOH	ethyl alcohol
EUA	examination under anesthesia
Exc	excision
expl	exploration
ext	external

F

F	Fahrenheit, degree of
FB	foreign body
FBS	fasting blood sugar

FDP	fibrinogen degradation products
Fe	iron
FEF	forced expiratory flow
$FeSO_4$	ferrous sulfate
FEV	forced expiratory volume
FEV1	1st second of expiration
FFA	free fatty acids
FH	fundal height
FHR	fetal heart rate
FHT	fetal heart tones
fib	fibrillation
fld ext	fluid extract
FRC	functional residual capacity
FSH	follicle-stimulating hormone
FTP	failure to progress
FTSG	full-thickness skin graft
FTT	failure to thrive
F/U	follow-up
FUO	fever of unknown origin
FVC	forced vital capacity
FWB	full weight bearing
fx	fracture

G

G	gravida
GA	general anesthesia
ga	gestational age
GB	gallbladder
GC	*Neisseria* gonorrhea
GE	gastroenteritis
gen	general
GET	general endotracheal intubation
GFR	glomerular filtration rate
GH	growth hormone
GI	gastrointestinal
g	gram
GME	graduate medical education
G-6-P	glucose-6-phosphate
G-6-PD	glucose-6-phosphate dehydrogenase
gr	grain
GSW	gunshot wound

GTT	glucose tolerance test
gtt	drop(s)
GU	genitourinary
GYN	gynecology

H

HA	headache
HA	hepatitis A
H/A	heated aerosol
HAA	hepatitis-associated antigen
HAL	hyperalimentation
Hb	hemoglobin
HB	heart block (1st, 2nd, or 3rd degree)
HB	hepatitis B
HbA_{1c}	hemoglobin A_{1c}, glycosylated hemoglobin A
HBAg	hepatitis B antigen
HBcAg	hepatitis B core antigen
HBeAg	hepatitis B e antigen
HBIG	hepatitis B immunoglobulin (also HBIg)
HBP	high blood pressure
HBsAb	hepatitis B surface antibody
HBsAg	hepatitis B surface antigen
HBV	hepatitis B virus
HCC	home care coordinator
hCG	human chorionic gonadotropin
HCl	hydrochloric acid
HCO_3	bicarbonate
Hct	hematocrit
HCTZ	hydrochlorothiazide
HCVD	hypertensive cardiovascular disease
HEENT	head/eyes/ears/nose/throat
HELLP	hemolysis, elevated liver enzymes, and low platelet count
H-flu	*haemophilus influenzae*
Hgb	hemoglobin
HGH	human growth hormone
H/H	hemoglobin/hematocrit
H/I	homicidal ideation
Histo	histoplasmosis
HIV	human immunodeficiency virus

HIVD	herniated interventricular disk
hm	hand motions
HMD	hyaline membrane disease
HNO_3	nitric acid
HNP	herniated nucleus pulposus
H_2O	water
H_2O_2	hydrogen peroxide
HO	house officer
HOB	head of bed
H&P	history and physical
hpf	high-power field
HPI	history of present illness
HR	heart rate
hr	hour
hs	at bedtime
H_2SO_4	sulfuric acid
Ht	height
HTN	hypertension
HVD	hypertensive vascular disease
HW	housewife
Hx	history
hyst	hysterectomy

I

I_{131}	radioactive iodine
IAM	internal auditory meatus
IBC	iron-binding capacity
IC	inspiratory capacity
ICBG	illiac crest bone graft
ICCP	intracapsular cataract pressure
ICF	intracellular fluid
ICU	intensive care unit
ID	intradermal
id	identification
I&D	incision and drainage
IDL	intraocular lens
IDU	idoxuridine
IFA	indirect fluorescent antibody
Ig	immunoglobulin
IgG	immunoglobulin G
IgM	immunoglobulin M

IHA	indirect hemagglutination
IHSS	idiopathic hypertrophic subaortic stenosis
IJ	ileojejunal
IM	intramuscular
IMF	inferior maxillary fracture
Imp	impression
IMV	intermittent mandatory ventilation
Ing	inguinal
INH	isoniazid
I&O	intake and output
IOCG	interoperative cholangiography
IOP	intraocular pressure
IP	intraperitoneal
ip	interim permitte
IPPB	intermittent positive pressure breathing
IRV	inspiratory reserve volume
IS	incentive spirometer
IT	intrathecal
ITP	immunologic thrombocytopenia
IU	international units
IUD	intrauterine device
IUG	intrauterine gestation
IUGR	intrauterine growth retardation
IUP	intrauterine pregnancy
IUT	intrauterine transfusion
IV	intravenous
IVH	intraventricular hemorrhage
IVP	intravenous pyelogram
IVPB	intravenous piggyback
IV push	intravenous push
IVS	intraventricular septum

J

JODM	juvenile-onset diabetes mellitus
JRA	juvenile rheumatoid arthritis
jt	joint
JVD	jugular venous distention
JVP	jugular venous pressure

K

K^+	potassium
KCl	potassium chloride

kg	kilogram
KP	keratic precipitates
KPE	kelmas phacoemulsification
KUB	kidneys, ureter, and bladder

L

L	liter
L1–L2	1st and 2nd lumbar vertebrae
LA	local anesthesia
LAC	long arm cast
LAD	left axis deviation
LAH	left axial hypertrophy
lap	laparotomy
LATS	long arm thumb spica
lb	pound
LB	lower back
LBBB	left bundle branch block
LBP	lower back pain
LBW	low birth weight
LC	living children
LCD	liquor carbonis detergens
LCS	lichen chronicus simplex
LD	lethal dose
LD_{50}	median lethal dose
LDH	lactic dehydrogenase
L-dopa	levodopa
LE	lupus erythematosus
le	left extremity
LFT	liver function test
lg	large
LGA	large for gestational age
LGL	Lown-Ganong-Levine
LH	luteinizing hormone
lig	ligation
lih	left inguinal hernia
liq	liquid
LL	left lung
LLC	long leg cast
LLE	left lower extremity
LLL	lower left lobe
LLQ	left lower quadrant
LMD	local medical doctor

LMP	last menstrual period
LOA	left occiput anterior
LOC	loss of consciousness
LOP	left occiput posterior
LOT	left occiput transverse
LP	lumbar puncture
LPT	licensed psychiatric technician
LR	Ringer's lactate
LS	lumbosacral
LSW	licensed social worker
LTB	laryngotracheobronchitis
LUD	left upper decubitus
LUE	left upper extremity
LUL	left upper lobe
LUQ	left upper quadrant
LVD	left ventricular dysfunction
LVET	left ventricular ejection time
LVH	left ventricular hypertrophy
LVID	left ventricular internal dimension
LVN	licensed vocational nurse
LVP	left ventricular pressure
L&W	living and well

M

m	meter
M/A	Mexican American
MA	mental age
MAV	minute alveolar volume
MCA	motorcycle accident
mca	middle cerebral artery
mcg	microgram
mch	mean corpuscular hemoglobin
MCH	Mission Community Hospital
MCHC	mean corpuscular hemoglobin count
MCP	metacarpophalangeal
MCV	mean corpuscular volume
M.D.	medical doctor
mEq	milliequivalents
MER	medical emergency room
met	metastasis
MG	myasthenia gravis

Mg^{++}	magnesium
mg/dl	milligram/deciliter
$Mg(OH)_2$	magnesium hydroxide
$MgSO_4$	magnesium sulfate
MH	mental health
MHC	mental health crisis
MI	myocardial infarction
MIC	minimal inhibitory concentration
mL	milliliter
ML	midline
MLH	Martin Luther Hospital
mm	millimeter
mm Hg	millimeters of mercury
MMR	maternal mortality rate
MMR	mumps, measles, rubella immunizations
MOA	monoamine oxidase
mod	moderate
MOM	milk of magnesia
MR	mitral regurgitation
MR__×	may repeat __ times
MRI	magnetic resonance imaging
MS	morphine sulfate
ms	mitral stenosis
MTX	methotrexate
MV	minute volume
mv	multivitamins
MVA	motor vehicle accident
MVP	mitral valve prolapse
MVV	maximal voluntary ventilation
MZ	monozygotic (twins)

N

Na^+	sodium
NA	nurse's aide
N/A	not applicable
NaCl	sodium chloride
NAD	no acute distress
$NaHCO_3$	sodium bicarbonate
NB	newborn
Neb meds	nebulized medications
NEC	necrotizing enterocolitis

neg	negative
NG	nasogastric
NH_4Cl	ammonium chloride
NIL	not in active labor
NICU	neonatal intensive care unit
NK	not known
NKA	no known allergies
nl	normal
NLP	no light perception
nm	neuromuscular
NMR	nuclear magnetic resonance
noc	night
NOS	not otherwise specified
NP	nasopharynx
NPC	near point of convergence
NPDR	nonproliferative diabetic retinopathy
NPH	neutral protamine Hagedorn (insulin)
NPN	nonprotein nitrogen
NPO	nil per os (nothing by mouth)
NS	normal saline
NSR	normal sinus rhythm
NST	nonstress test
NSVD	normal spontaneous vaginal delivery
NT	nasotracheal
NTG	nitroglycerin
N&V	nausea and vomiting

O

O	negative
O_2	oxygen
OA	occiput anterior
OB	obstetric
OB+	occult blood positive
OBS	organic brain syndrome
OCG	oral cholecystogram
OCP	oral contraceptive pills
OCT	oxytocin challenge test
o.d.	right eye
OD	overdose
OM	otitis media
OMFS	oral and maxillofacial surgery

OOB	out of bed
OOP	out of plaster
op	operation
OP	occiput posterior
OPC	outpatient clinic
OPD	outpatient department
OPV	oral poliovirus vaccine
OR	operating room
ORIF	open reduction and internal fixation
o.s.	left eye
osm	osmolar
OT	occupational therapy
otc	over the counter
o.u.	each eye, both eyes
oz	ounce

P

P	pulse
$\bar{p}$	after
p	pressure
PA	pernicious anemia
pa	posteroanterior
P&A	percussion and auscultation
PAC	premature atrial contractions
PAP	Papanicolaou smear
Par	paranoid
Para I	primipara
PARR	post anesthesia recovery room
PAS	para-aminosalicylic acid
PAT	paroxysmal atrial tachycardia
path	pathology
Pb	barometric pressure
Pb	phenobarbital
PB	piggyback
PBI	protein-bound iodine
pc	after meals
PCC	patient care coordinator
PCN	penicillin
P_{CO_2}	partial pressure of carbon dioxide
PCWP	pulmonary capillary wedge pressure
PD	interpupillary distance

PDA	patent ductus arteriosus
PD&P	postural drainage and percussion
PDR	Physicians' Desk Reference
PE	physical examination
PE	pulmonary embolus
PEAU	psychiatric emergency admitting unit
Ped	pediatrician
Peds	pediatrics
PEEP	positive end-expiratory pressure
PEFR	peak expiratory flow rate
PEP	peak expiratory pressure
perf	perforation
PERLA	pupils equal, reactive to light and accommodation
PERRLA	pupils equal, round, reactive to light and accommodation
PET	positron emission tomography
PETs	pressure equalization tubes
PEU	protected environment unit
PFR	peak flow rate
PFT	pulmonary function test
Pg	pregnant
1° PG	one hour postglucola
pH	relationship between hydrogen ion concentration of a sample solution to a standard solution (pH 7 = neutral; pH <7 = acidic; pH >7= alkaline)
PH	past history
PHA	phytohemagglutinin
PharmD	Doctor of Pharmacy
PhD	Doctor of Philosophy
PHN	public health nurse
P/I	paranoid ideation
PI	present illness
PICU	pediatric intensive care unit
PID	pelvic inflammatory disease
PIH	pregnancy-induced hypertension
PIP	proximal interphalangeal (joint)
PK	psychokinesis
PKU	phenylketonuria
PL	pediatric level
PMD	private medical doctor
PMH	past medical history
PMI	point of maximal impulse

PMP	previous menstrual period
PM&R	physical medicine and rehabilitation
PNB	prostatic needle biopsy
PND	paroxysmal nocturnal dyspnea
PNM	perinatal mortality
PNMR	perinatal mortality rate
PO	postoperative
po	per os (by mouth)
Po_2	partial pressure of oxygen
post	posterior
Postop	postoperative
POV	privately owned vehicle
pp	postpartum
PP	postprandial
PPD	purified protein derivative (tuberculin)
Ppeak	postoperative peak pressure
PPP	palatopharyngoplasty
PR	per rectum
PRBC	packed red blood cells
preg	pregnancy
preop	preoperative
prep	preparation
prn	whenever necessary
prob	problem
prog	prognosis
PROM	premature rupture of membranes
Protime (PT)	prothrombin time
prox	proximal
PS	pulmonary stenosis
PSP	phenolsulfonphthalein
Pstat	static pressure
pt	patient
PT	physical therapy
PT	prothrombin time
PTA	prior to admission
PTB	patella tendon bearing
PTH	parathyroid hormone
PTL	preterm labor
PTT	partial thromboplastin time
PTU	propylthiouracil
PUBS	percutaneous umbilical vein blood sampling
PUD	peptic ulcer disease

PVC	premature ventricular contractions
PWB	partial weight bearing
px	pneumothorax
PX	physical examination
PZI	protamine zinc insulin

Q

q	every (e.g., q8h)
qam	every morning
qd	every day or once a day
qh	every hour
qhs	every night at bedtime
qid	four times a day
qod	every other day
qs	quantity sufficient to make

R

R	respiration
ra	room air
RA	rheumatoid arthritis
RAD	right axis deviation
RAE	right atrial enlargement
RAF	rheumatoid arthritis factor
RAH	right atrial hypertrophy
RAI	radioactive iodine
RAIU	radioactive iodine uptake
RAO	right anterior oblique
RAP	right atrial pressure
RAS	renal artery stenosis
RBBB	right bundle branch block
rbc	red blood cell
RBC	red blood count
RBF	renal blood flow
RCA	right coronary artery
RCD	relative cardiac dullness
RCS	reticulum cell sarcoma
RD	respiratory disease
RDA	recommended daily allowance
rda	right dorsoanterior
rdp	right dorsoposterior
RDS	respiratory distress syndrome

RE	regional enteritis
re	right extremity
rehab	rehabilitation
req	request
retic	reticulocyte
RFS	renal function study
Rh	Rhesus (factor)
RHD	rheumatic heart disease
RI	respiratory illness
RIA	radioimmunoassay
RICU	Respiratory Intensive Care Unit
RJ	Robert Jones dressing
RL	right lung
RLC	residual lung capacity
RLE	right lower extremity
RLF	retrolental fibroplasia
RLL	right lower lobe
RLQ	right lower quadrant
RML	right middle lobe
RN	registered nurse
RND	radical neck dissection
R/O	rule out
ROA	right occiput anterior
ROAD	reversible obstructive artery disease
ROM	range of motion
rom	rupture of membranes
ROP	right occiput posterior
ROS	review of systems
ROT	right occiput transverse
RPR	rapid plasma reagin (syphilis screen)
rpr	reactive protein reagent
RQ	respiratory quotient
RR	recovery room
rr	respiratory rate
RRR	regular rate and rhythm
R/S	restraint and seclusion
RSR	regular sinus rhythm
Rt	right
RT	radiation therapy
RTA	renal tubular acidosis
RTC	return to clinic
RTO	return to office

RUE	right upper extremity
RUL	right upper lobe
RUQ	right upper quadrant
RV	residual volume
RVE	right ventricular enlargement
RVID	right ventricular internal dimension
RVT	renal vein thrombosis
Rx	prescription
rx	treatment, therapy

S

s̄	without
S1 & S2	heart sounds, first and second
S3 & S4	heart sounds, third and fourth
S/A	suicide attempt
S&A	sugar and acetone
SAB	spontaneous abortion
SAC	short arm cast
SAH	subarachnoid hemorrhage
SAP	systemic arterial pressure
sat	saturated
SATS	short arm thumb spica
SB	standby
SBE	subacute bacterial endocarditis
SBO	small bowel obstruction
SCUT	schizophrenia, chronic undifferentiated type
SE	southeast
SEM	systolic ejection murmur
SG	Swan-Ganz
SG	specific gravity
SGA	small for gestational age
SGOT	serum glutamic-oxaloacetic transaminase (ASP)
SGPT	serum glutamic pyruvic transaminase (ALT)
SIADH	syndrome inappropriate secretion of antidiuretic hormone
sig	let it be labeled, write
SIMV	synchronized intermittent mandatory ventilation
SL	sublingual
SLC	short leg cast
SLE	systemic lupus erythematosus
SLWC	short leg walking cast

SMR	submucosal resection
SNF	skilled nursing facility
S&O	salpingo-oophorectomy
SO_1	oxygen saturation
SOAP	subjective, objective assessment plan
SOAPE	subjective, objective assessment plan, evaluation
sob	side of bed
SOB	shortness of breath
sol	solution
SOM	serous otitis media
sos	if necessary
S/P	status post
SPA	salt-poor albumin
spec	specimen
SPECT	single photon emission computed tomography
SPT	senior psychiatric technician
SQ	subcutaneous
SR	sedimentation rate
SROM	spontaneous rupture of membranes
ss	one half
SSE	soap suds enema
SSE	sterile speculum examination
SSKI	saturated solution potassium iodide
SSS	sick sinus syndrome
S/T	suicide ideation
stat	immediately
STSG	split-thickness skin graft
suct	suction
SUN	serum urea nitrogen
supp	suppository
SV	supraventricular
sx	symptoms
syr	syrup

T

T	temperature
T1, T2	first, second thoracic vertebrae
T3	triiodothyronine
T4	thyroxine
TA	trained aid
T&A	tonsillectomy and adenoidectomy

tab	tablet
TAB	therapeutic abortion
TAH	total abdominal hysterectomy
TAL	tendon Achilles lengthening
TAT	tetanus antitoxin
TB	tuberculosis
tbsp	tablespoon
TBW	total body water
tc	total capacity
TC	temporary custody
T&C	type and crossmatch
TCDB	turn, cough, deep breathe
TCI	transient cerebral ischemia
TCN	tetracycline
Td	tetanus and diphtheria toxins
TEF	tracheoesophageal fistula
TGT	thromboplastin generation test
T&H	type and hold
TIA	transient ischemic attack
TIBC	total iron-binding capacity
tid	*ter in die* (three times a day)
TIE	transient ischemic episode
TKO	to keep open
TL	tubal ligation
TLC	tender loving care
tlc	total lung capacity
tm	temporomandibular
TM	tympanic membrane
tmj	temporomandibular joint
TMP/SMX	trimethoprim-sulfamethoxazole
TMST	treadmill stress test
TND	term normal delivery
TO	telephone order
TOA	tubo-ovarian abscess
toco	tocodynamometer
TPN	total parenteral nutrition
TPR	temperature, pulse, and respiration
TR	tricuspid regurgitation
Tr	trace
tr	tincture
TRC	therapeutic residential center

Trend	Trendelenburg
TRIS	tris(hydroxymethyl)aminomethane
TS	tricuspid stenosis
TSH	thyroid-stimulating hormone
tsp	teaspoon
TTN	transient tachypnea of newborn
TURB	transurethral resection of the bladder
TURBT	transurethral resection of the bladder tumor
TURP	transurethral resection of the prostate
TV	tidal volume
TVC	total volume capacity
TVH	total vaginal hysterectomy
TWE	tap water enema
Tx	treatment

U

U	unit
UA	uric acid
UA	urinalysis
UC	uterine contractions
UCHD	usual childhood diseases
UCHI	usual childhood illnesses
UCI(MC)	University of California, Irvine (Medical Center)
ud	as directed
UGI	upper gastrointestinal
UL	upper lobe
U&L	upper and lower
ULQ	upper left quadrant
UMB	umbilicus
UMN	upper motor neuron
UMNB	upper motor neurogenic bladder
UN	urea nitrogen
ung	ointment
uni	one
U/O	urinary output
UOQ	upper outer quadrant
UPJ	ureteropelvic junction
URD	upper respiratory disease
URI	upper respiratory infection
Urol	urology

URQ	upper right quadrant
U/S	sonogram (ultrasound)
UTI	urinary tract infection
UVJ	ureterovesical junction

V

V	ventricular
v	venous
VA	ventriculoatrial
Va	visual acuity
Vac̄ C	visual acuity with correction
Vac C	visual acuity without correction
vasc	vascular
VB	viable birth
VC	vital capacity
VCG	vector cardiogram
VCR	vincristine
VCUG	voiding cystourethrogram
Vds	volume of dead space
VD	venereal disease
VDRL	Venereal Disease Research Laboratories (syphilis screen)
VE	vaginal examination
Ve vent	expired gas volume ventilator
VF	ventricular fibrillation
vf	visual field
VH	ventricular hypertrophy
V/H	visual hallucinations
Vits	vitamins
VMA	vanillylmandelic acid
VNA	Visiting Nurses Association
VO	verbal order
vol	volume
VP	vasa previa
VP	ventriculoperitoneal
V&P	vagotomy and pyloroplasty
VPC	ventricular premature contractions
VS	vital signs
VSD	ventricular septal defect
Vt	tidal volume
Vtx	vertex

W

W	weakly positive
Warming Blk	hypothermia mattress
W/B	waist belt
WBC	white blood cells, white blood cell count
WBTT	weight bearing to tolerance
W/C	wheelchair
WD/WN	well developed/well nourished
WNL	within normal limits
WO	without
WPF	Wright peak flow
WR	Wassermann reaction
wr	weakly reactive
wt	weight
w/u	workup

X

x	mean value
×	times
X^1	exophoria (near)
XM	crossmatch
XR	x-ray
XT	exotrophia (distance)
X(T)	intermittent exotropia (distance)
XT^I	exotropia (near)

Y

y	year
yo	years old
yo	years of
YS	yellow spot (retina)

Z

Z	zero
ZIG	zoster immune globulin
Zno	zinc oxide

APPENDIX Y: USEFUL PHONE NUMBERS

Hospital

- Information ________________
- Paging ________________
- **Labs**
  - Arterial Blood Gas Lab ________________
  - Blood Bank ________________
  - Chemistry ________________
  - Hematology ________________
  - Microbiology ________________
  - Special Chemistry ________________
- **Services**
  - Center for Fetal Evaluation ________________
  - Genetics
    - Counseling ________________
    - Lab ________________
  - Medical Social Work ________________
- **Wards**
  - Antepartum ________________
  - Labor and Delivery ________________
  - Postpartum ________________
- **Physician Consult**
  - Cardiology ________________
  - Infectious Disease ________________
  - Internal Medicine ________________
  - Neurology ________________
  - Perinatology ________________
  - Surgery ________________

INDEX

D

E

F

I

J

K

L